DRUGS AND NUTRITION
IN THE GERIATRIC PATIENT

CONTEMPORARY ISSUES IN CLINICAL NUTRITION
VOLUME 7

SERIES EDITOR

Richard S. Rivlin, M.D.

EDITORIAL ADVISORY BOARD

Myron Brin, Ph.D.

Leon Ellenbogen, Ph.D.

Elaine B. Feldman, M.D.

Sami A. Hashim, M.D.

Sheldon Konigsberg, M.D.

Also in the Series

DRUGS AND NUTRITION IN THE GERIATRIC PATIENT

Edited by

Daphne A. Roe, M.D.

Professor of Nutrition
Division of Nutritional Sciences
Cornell University
Ithaca, New York

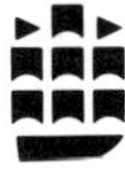

CHURCHILL LIVINGSTONE
NEW YORK, EDINBURGH, LONDON, AND MELBOURNE
1984

Distributed in the United Kingdom by Churchill Livingstone,
Robert Stevenson House, 1–3 Baxter Place, Leith Walk,
Edinburgh EH1 3AF and associated companies, branches
and representatives throughout the world.

First published in 1984
Printed in U.S.A.

ISBN 0-443-08218-9
9 8 7 6 5 4 3 2 1

Library of Congress Cataloging in Publication Data
Main entry under title:

Drugs and nutrition in the geriatric patient.

   (Contemporary issues in clinical nutrition; v. 7)
   Bibliography: p.
   Includes index.
   Contents: Drug usage by the elderly / Dennis E.
Hyams — Food choices of the elderly / Eleanor D.
Schlenker—Food effects on drug absorption in the
elderly / C.T. Viswanathan and Peter G. Welling—[etc.]
   1. Aged—Diseases—Addresses, essays, lectures.
2. Drugs and the aged—Addresses, essays, lectures.
3. Aged—Nutrition—Addresses, essays, lectures.
I. Roe, Daphne A. II. Series. [DNLM: 1. Drug Therapy—
—Adverse effects. 2. Drug Therapy—In old age.
3. Nutrition Disorders—Chemically induced. 4. Nutrition
disorders—In old age. W 1 CO769MQH v. 7 / WD 100 D794]
RC952.5.D78 1984   615′.7′0880565   83-20872
ISBN 0-443-08218-9

Manufactured in the United States of America

Contributors

Barry Cusack, M.D.
Senior Registrar in Geriatrics
Northwick Park Hospital and
Clinical Research Center
Harrow, Middlesex
England

Michael J. Denham, M.D.
Consulting Physician in Geriatric Medicine
Northwick Park Hospital and Clinical Research Center
Harrow, Middlesex
England

Dennis E. Hyams, M.B., F.R.C.P. (CLON)
Senior Medical Director
Merck Sharpe & Dohme International
Rahway, New Jersey

Daphne A. Roe, M.D.
Professor of Nutrition
Division of Nutritional Sciences
Cornell University
Ithaca, New York

Eleanor D. Schlenker, Ph.D.
Associate Professor and Chairperson
Department of Human Nutrition and Foods
College of Agriculture
Unversity of Vermont
Burlington, Vermont

C.T. Viswanathan, Ph.D.
Biopharmaceutics Division
Food and Drug Administration
Rockville, Maryland

Peter G. Welling, D.Sc.
Professor
School of Pharmacy
University of Wisconsin
Madison, Wisconsin

Foreword

The intent of a physician to benefit his patient is no safeguard against injury of his patient; if it were, there would be no iatrogenic diseases.

Iatrogenic diseases, "conditions induced by a physician," historically have resulted from a host of potent agents and mixtures administered by physicians to the limits of tolerance or to a level of intoxication, from other "therapeutic" measures in the past such as blood-letting or the mistaken use of dietary restrictions. Such effects usually were acute in nature because of the relatively brief periods during which these heroic measures were prescribed.

Sagacious observers warned early against many of these common practices. For example, Robert Burton, in *The Anatomy of Melancholy* (1660 edition) quotes Arnoldus: "A wise physician will not give physick, but upon necessity, and first try medicinal diet, before he proceeds to medicinall cure." Cicero likewise recognized that: "A careful physician . . . before he attempts to administer a remedy to his patient, must investigate not only the malady of the man . . . but also his habits when in health, and his physical constitution."

Today's therapeutic regimens comprise highly effective pharmacologic agents, selected and designed as metabolic alterants, hence as agents that often may change the absorption, transport, metabolism, excretion, or cellular function of a nutrient. Modern surgical procedures similarly may alter drastically the nutrient intake, absorptive or excretory capabilities, or metabolic processes. Today, such measures frequently are long-term chronic therapies that may be even of lifelong duration, e.g., antidiabetic agents, systemic contraceptives, cardiovascular drugs, psychopharmacologic agents, ambulatory TPN, renal dialysis, to note but a few of the most common.

These have profound implications for the nutriture of the patient . . . implications which, if not appropriately recognized and managed, result in iatrogenic disease or disaster.

Nutritional considerations are, therefore, a significant part of the design of modern therapeutic regimens, for as Hippocrates observed, ". . . the art of medicine would not have been invented at first, nor would it have been a subject of investigation (for there would be no need of it), if when men were indisposed the same food and other articles of regimen which they eat and drink when in good health were proper for them, and if no others were preferable to these. But now necessity itself made medicine to be sought out and discovered by men, since the same things when administered to the sick, which agreed with them when in good health, neither did nor do agree with them . . .''

Understanding of the nutritional implications of drugs and application of this knowledge are requisites for today's "wise physician." He may not under all therapeutic regimens follow Hippocrates' aphorism ". . . old men have little heat in them, therefore they require but little food. For much nourishment extinguishes that heat."

William J. Darby, M.D., Ph.D.
Vanderbilt University
School of Medicine

Preface

The elderly are the chief drug users in our society. Whereas older people may require drugs for treatment of acute or chronic health problems, their tolerance for drugs may be less than that of younger people. Age is known to alter drug disposition, but in the elderly observed changes in drug absorption, metabolism, or elimination may be due to diet or nutrition. Further, elderly people who are on long-term or multiple drug therapies may be at risk for development of drug-induced malnutrition. This book addresses the diets of the elderly, their intakes of prescription and OTC drugs, and the interactive effects of aging, diet and nutrition as factors which explain untoward effects of drugs in the elderly.

The book is intended for physicians and other health professionals who are concerned with geriatric care.

As Editor, I would like to express my thanks to the editorial staff of Churchill Livingstone, especially Gene Kearn, and also to my secretary, Beverly Hastings, for her invaluable assistance.

Daphne A. Roe, M.D.

Contents

1 | Drug Usage by the Elderly

Dennis E. Hyams

The increasing numbers and proportion of elderly persons in developed countries during the 20th century is now a well-recognized phenomenon. The proportion of elderly over the age of 65 years is reaching 15% or more in some European countries; in the United States, the figure is now 11%.[1] These percentages will continue to increase during the remainder of this century, and it is projected that in the United Kingdom the proportion of the very old (aged 85 and over) will increase at the fastest rate of all. The implications of these demographic trends are very significant in regard to the cost (in money and work force) of the delivery of health care to nations, and to the pattern of prescription and consumption of drugs.

This chapter sets out to examine patterns of drug usage in the elderly, with particular emphasis on the United States and Europe. In some populations, the proportion of elderly persons (aged 60 years and over) is very high (about 20%); in these populations, at least 50% of the total drug consumption is by the elderly.[2] By the more usual definition of *elderly* as 65 years and over, in the fiscal year 1976 the elderly (then 10% of the population) accounted for 25% of the national United States expenditure on drugs and drug sundries (totaling $11.2 billion). In that year, each elderly person spent an average of over $100 for prescribed and over-the-counter (OTC) drugs.[3] In the United Kingdom, the elderly represent 13% of the population but are the recipients of nearly one third of National Health Service expenditure on drug prescriptions.[4] Although the definition of *elderly* is open to discussion, there is meaning in adopting the age of 65 years as a dividing line between "middle" and "old" age: it has been shown that in the United States, nearly 40% of persons over 65 years of age have some restriction of major activities.[5]

1

Systematic epidemiological studies on drug use, misuse, and abuse in large elderly populations are not yet available, although the literature contains many individual reports concerning such usage in institutions and in the home. These reports will be considered in more detail later, together with an analysis of drug usage in the elderly by the frequency of prescription of various drug groups. Here some general principles will be considered concerning patterns of disease and treatment in old age.

Senescence is characterized by lack of physiological reserves, facilitating disturbances of homeostasis in elderly persons. Multiple pathology is the rule in old age and this phenomenon not only makes accurate diagnosis more difficult (a problem compounded by the frequently atypical presentation of illness in old age) but also leads to polypharmacy.

EXTENT OF DRUG USAGE IN THE ELDERLY

Many elderly patients living at home take three or more different drugs daily;[6-9] in institutions, the quantity frequently increases to five to ten different drugs per day or even more.[10,11]

Not surprisingly, the incidence of adverse drug reactions increases in old age, although it is difficult to assess the true incidence because the published studies vary in design and statistical validity.[12] Several reports suggest that adverse reactions are two to three times as common after the age of 60 years as prior to this age.[13-15] The incidence also rises abruptly in patients taking five to six or more drugs daily.[11,14,16] There is also a sex difference in the incidence of adverse drug reactions in the elderly: women are affected more often than men.[13,15] Adverse drug reactions appear to be particularly common in the United States.[17] The reasons for these increases in drug reactions in old age are several—not just polypharmacy itself, but also medication errors (more likely because of multiple drugs, complicated regimens, and factors related to patient compliance) and altered pharmacokinetics and pharmacodyamics in the elderly.[18-24]

With regard to patterns of illness and type of therapy, it is well established that cardiovascular disorders are the commonest ailments of old age, leading to widespread and often prolonged use of diuretics, digitalis glycosides, and other forms of cardiac therapy; other conditions include arthritides (anti-inflammatory and analgesic drugs), psychic disturbances (psycholeptics and cerebroactive agents), and respiratory and gastrointestinal conditions. Of particular interest is the widespread use of antihypertensive agents (including beta blockers) in this age group in the United Kingdom; the definition and management of hypertension in the elderly are topics of continuing controversy, and the elderly do not always tolerate beta blocker therapy well. Despite these patterns of illness, the actual prescription rates of various drug groups may be different from those expected from the frequency of types of disease.

These observations lead naturally to the classification of drugs used in the elderly, as suggested by T. N. Rudd, M.D., of Southampton many years ago:

Group 1. Useless drugs
Group 2. Inappropriate drugs
Group 3. Potentially dangerous drugs

Much iatrogenic illness could be avoided if physicians were more alert to these categories. "Useless" drugs are, for example, antiaging remedies; "inappropriate" drugs are drugs given unnecessarily (a common error in treating the elderly—especially when the prescription of a drug is continued uncritically over many months or even years, as is often the case with diuretics and digitalis). All other drugs fall into group 3.

PATTERNS OF DRUG USAGE BY THE ELDERLY

This section will consider several published surveys of drug use by the elderly, at home and in various types of institution, and recent unpublished figures from an international audit of prescribing in general practice.

The Elderly at Home

Published Surveys Inevitably, most surveys of prescribing for patients in the community rely on data obtained from prescriptions after the drug has been dispensed by the pharmacist; errors arise in interpretation because little or no account is taken of the clinical situation or of patient compliance.

Law and Chalmers[6] reported on all patients aged 75 and over in a single general practice in London (150 patients in all). Eighty-seven percent were taking drugs regularly, a figure three times that of the general population; 34% were taking three or more different drugs every day, the commonest being analgesics, psychotropic drugs, genitourinary drugs, and cardiac drugs (diuretics and digitalis).

Shaw and Opit[7] found that half the patients aged 70 and over in a Birmingham, England, general practice were on long-term drug therapy, mainly for heart disease, depression, and anxiety. Fourteen percent had not been in contact with their general practitioners for six months or longer, providing an index of "repeat prescribing" by doctors without seeing the patient—a practice also very common in the United States, where telephone consultations are more frequent than in England. This study, although widely quoted, was criticized by Crombie et al.,[25] but the desirability of careful review before represcribing any drug for the elderly had been emphasized by Forbes,[26] who also indicated that "inherited therapy" is common; i.e., a drug started in middle age may be considered unsuitable for the elderly, but the patient may resist any change to a more appropriate drug. Sometimes long-standing prescriptions for a particular drug are knowingly continued into old age without the physician being aware of the undesirability of the drug in the elderly. Clearly the solution to both these problems lies in further education of both patient and physician.

Manasse[27] reported that almost a quarter of 1,133 requests for repeat prescriptions came from patients aged 65 and over. Analyses of repeat prescribing for the elderly in their own practices have been reported by Dawson[28] in Sussex, England, and Tulloch[29] in Oxford, England. Dawson found an incidence of 60% of repeat prescriptions in 99 patients aged over 79 years, and Tulloch reported an incidence of 48% in 175 patients aged 65 or over. In the latter study, 12% more women than men received repeat prescriptions and for both sexes the incidence increased with age over 65—a phenomenon that is well recognized. Over 44% of the repeats in Tulloch's study were for cardiovascular and central nervous system disorders (in almost equal numbers). More important, only 62% of the drugs prescribed were considered by Tulloch to be really necessary: 10% were clearly not needed, and 28% were "equivocal." One third of the unnecessary drugs were psychotropics (tranquilizers, hypnotics, and antidepressants in almost equal numbers), but cardiovascular drugs came a close second.

This study calls to mind several others that point to unnecessary long-term medication in the elderly. Gibson and O'Hare[30] and Dall[31] considered that two thirds to three quarters of the elderly patients they studied were taking digitalis or digoxin unnecessarily. Later studies confirmed that withdrawal of chronic digoxin treatment need have no adverse effect in regard to the development of congestive heart failure.[32-34] The value of long-term diuretic therapy in the elderly has been called into question by the studies of Burr et al.[35] in the United Kingdom and Myers et al.[36] in Canada. In Sweden, it has been reported that iron tablets are widely overprescribed, especially for the elderly.[37] Further discussion of unnecessary repeat prescribing is given in the section on the elderly in long-term care (see below and Bruce[38]).

In Nordic countries generally, the use of medicines increases with age; for patients over 65 years, more than ten times as many prescriptions are written as for the age group 15 to 35 years.[39] In Sweden, cardiovascular drugs are the commonest group prescribed after 60 years of age.[40]

In the United States, it was reported in 1968 that diazepam, chlordiazepoxide, and propoxyphene were the most commonly prescribed drugs for the elderly.[41] In a later community-based survey,[42] the most frequently used drugs in the over-60 population were analgesics, followed (at a distance) by cardiovascular drugs, laxatives, vitamins, antacids, and antianxiety agents. In a similar study, however, it was reported that cardiovascular drugs represented over 60% of prescriptions for the elderly in Washington, D.C.[43]

Freeman[44] reported that in a Health Care practice in Southampton, England, cardiovascular drugs (including diuretics) were those most often prescribed, followed by analgesics and psychotropics. Observations on analgesic use in the elderly were made by Stewart et al.,[45] and on psychotherapeutic drugs in a report from the U.S. National Institute on Drug Abuse.[46] The latter emphasizes the vulnerability of the elderly to psychotherapeutic drug misuse and abuse.

The literature on prescribing for the elderly in general practice was reviewed by Knox.[47] The epidemiological study from Oxford by Skegg et al.[48] showed the relationship between multiple-drug therapy and age; at all ages, a higher proportion of women than men received drugs. Similar findings were reported from a geriatric screening clinic in Florida by May et al.[49] Special problems may arise when an elderly patient comes home from the hospital with recommendations for medication. These problems are discussed in the section on compliance.

Unpublished Data from IMS International Unpublished data from an IMS International audit of prescribing in European general practices in 1981 is presented in Tables 1-1–1-5. The countries included in these tables are the United Kingdom, Germany, the Netherlands, and Belgium, respectively; Table 1-5 compares data from all four of these countries.

Each of the first four tables sets out a list of the 15 most prescribed categories of drugs in the country under consideration. The entries are ranked, however, according to the degree to which each is prescribed for patients aged 65 and over. In addition, some other groups are appended that have a major use in the elderly.

Table 1-1 shows, as anticipated, the importance of cardiac therapy, diuretics, and antirheumatics in geriatric therapeutics in the United Kingdom, but also shows the popularity of antihypertensives and beta blockers among physicians treating this age group. Table 1-2 shows that in Germany the drugs most used for the elderly are peripheral vasodilators (including use as putative cerebral vasodilators, an indication now less favored in many other European countries and in the United States). A close second is the antihypertensives—even more popular than in the

Table 1-1. Fifteen Most Prescribed Therapeutic Classes of Drugs, United Kingdom, 1981 (ranked according to proportionate use, within each therapeutic class, in subjects aged 65 years or over)

Therapeutic Class[a]	Percent Prescriptions for Patients $\geq$ 65 Years
Cardiac therapy	68.3
Diuretics	59.6
Antihypertensives[b]	52.7
Antirheumatics	42.7
Beta blockers[b]	42.0
Antiemetics	41.2
Psycholeptics	38.3
Antacids, antiflatulents, and anti–peptic ulcer drugs[c]	37.8
Analgesics[c]	34.6
Antiasthmatics	30.3
Psychoanaleptics	26.7
Antianemics	24.8
Topical corticosteroids	21.4
Cough and cold preparations[c]	20.5
Systemic antibiotics	12.8
Additional drugs with major use in the elderly:	
Peripheral vasodilators	68
Laxatives[c]	56
Cholagogues	42
Vitamins[c]	40
Vasoprotective drugs	29
Sex hormones	1

[a] See Table 1-5 for subgroups.
[b] Note relatively large usage in elderly patients.
[c] Prescribed use reflects only a fraction of total use because of large volume of over-the-counter sales.
Data by courtesy of IMS International, Inc.

United Kingdom. Cardiac and diuretic therapies are also much used. Two entries deserve special mention: topical antirheumatic preparations and vasoprotective drugs are important weapons of the therapeutic armamentarium of Germany. In the Netherlands (Table 1-3), cardiac and diuretic therapies take pride of place; one third of prescriptions for beta blockers are for elderly patients, but other antihypertensive agents are not represented in the most prescribed classes of drugs. Belgium (Table 1-4) shows similarities in these respects, but, like Germany, the most frequently prescribed drugs for the elderly are peripheral vasodilators.

Table 1-5 gives breakdowns of the therapeutic categories used in the first four tables and provides comparisons between the four countries under consideration. Some notable points will be made:

Rauwolfia, now rarely used in the United Kingdom, is mainly prescribed for the elderly, presumably in low dosage to avoid depression as a side effect. Ten times as many prescriptions (approximately 1.5 million) are written for Rauwolfia preparations in Germany as in the United Kingdom. Rauwolfia is relatively little used in the Netherlands.

There is widespread use of synthetic antihypertensive agents in all four countries, with a little over half the prescriptions being written for the elderly. Combina-

Table 1-2. Fifteen Most Prescribed Therapeutic Classes of Drugs, Germany, 1981 (ranked according to proportionate use, within each therapeutic class, in subjects aged 65 years or over)

Therapeutic Class	Percent Prescriptions for Patients ≥ 65 Years
Peripheral vasodilators	67.1
Antihypertensives[a]	64.0
Cardiac therapy	58.9
Vasoprotective drugs	41.9
Psycholeptics	40.7
Antirheumatics (topical)[b]	36.9
Antirheumatics (systemic)	36.3
Antacids, antiflatulents, and anti–peptic ulcer drugs[c]	27.4
Topical corticosteroids	24.1
Other therapeutic products[d]	22.6
Analgesics[c]	21.8
Cough and cold preparations[c]	17.8
Pharyngeal preparations[c]	12.6
Nasal decongestants[c]	10.5
Sex hormones	2.9
Additional drugs with major use in the elderly:	
Diuretics	57
Laxatives[c]	44
Psychoanaleptics	40
Cholagogues	40
Beta blockers	31
Vitamins[c]	25
Systemic antibiotics	12

[a] Note widespread use in elderly patients.
[b] Note popularity of topical antirheumatic preparations.
[c] Prescribed use reflects only a fraction of total use because of large volume of over-the-counter sales.
[d] A miscellaneous group of combination products.
Data by courtesy of IMS International, Inc.

tions including diuretics are used mainly for elderly patients in the United Kingdom and Germany. In both countries, two thirds of all prescriptions for this subclass of hypertensives are provided for the elderly.

Beta blockers are more popular in the United Kingdom than in the other three countries and are used in combination rarely in Belgium and to a modest extent in the United Kingdom, Germany, and the Netherlands.

The pattern of prescription of cardiac drugs is similar in all four countries, except for the predilection for cardiac and respiratory stimulants noted in the United Kingdom. However, the actual number of prescriptions in this category is relatively small.

Antirheumatics (excluding topicals) are prescribed more often in the United Kingdom than in the other countries; when topicals are included, Germany takes the lead.

The United Kingdom outstrips the other three countries in regard to the proportion of non-narcotic analgesics, antacids/antiflatulents/anti-peptic drugs, and laxatives prescribed for the elderly.

Netherlands and Belgium show low figures for cough and cold preparations, as compared to Germany, and especially to the United Kingdom. The use of anti-infective drugs in this clinical situation is considerable in the United Kingdom but appears to be negligible in the other three countries.

Psychoactive drugs—mood-elevating and mood-lowering—are less utilized for the elderly in the Netherlands than in the other countries. The use of neurotropics in the United Kingdom is not common but is mainly for the elderly; in Germany and Belgium, there is greater usage of these drugs, but one third of the prescriptions are for the under-65 population, whereas in the Netherlands over half

Table 1-3. Fifteen Most Prescribed Therapeutic Classes of Drugs, Netherlands, 1981 (ranked according to proportionate use, within each therapeutic class, in subjects aged 65 years or over)

Therapeutic Class	Percent Prescriptions for Patients ≥ 65 Years
Cardiac therapy	59.6
Diuretics	51.0
Antacids, antiflatulents, and anti–peptic ulcer drugs[a]	43.7
Beta blockers	33.6
Vitamins[a]	29.0
Antiasthmatics	26.8
Psycholeptics	25.9
Antirheumatics	24.5
Cough and cold preparations[a]	15.3
Analgesics[a]	15.1
Topical corticosteroids	14.8
Systemic antibiotics	12.1
Systemic antihistamines	11.4
Nasal decongestants[a]	4.4
Sex hormones	1.6
Additional drugs with major use in the elderly:	
Laxatives[a]	41

[a] Prescribed use reflects only a fraction of total use because of large volume of over-the-counter sales. Data by courtesy of IMS International, Inc.

the prescriptions are for the under-65 population.

It will be noted that vitamins—particularly vitamin A and D combinations and multivitamin mineral combinations—are prescribed for the elderly in the United Kingdom more than in the other countries.

The Elderly in Institutions

Long-Term Care (Residential Homes and Long-Term Hospitals) Many studies have appeared during the last 15 years or so. According to Cape,[9] similar patterns of drug use are to be found in long-term care facilities in Canada, Europe, and Australia. As in acute hospitals, polypharmacy is widespread, but the pattern of prescribing in long-term care facilities is different from that in acute hospitals, as would be expected. Although individual studies show differences in detail, it is apparent that the drugs most frequently used in long-term institutional settings are psychoactive drugs (including hypnotics), analgesics, and laxatives.

Prien and Caffey[50] surveyed 12 Veterans Administration hospitals in the United States and reviewed 2,682 patients aged 60 years and over. Seven hundred and eighteen patients (27%) had a primary diagnosis of organic brain syndrome; most also had other major diagnoses, since multiple pathology is the rule in the elderly. Ninety-four percent of the patients received medication (2,390 drugs, 77% classed as somatic [1,850 drugs], 19% as psychotherapeutic [464 drugs], and 3% as cognitive agents [76 drugs]). The commonest drugs were laxatives (35%), digoxin (16%), and thioridazine (15%). Individual wards and hospitals showed significant differences in prescribing patterns.

It is worth noting that psychotherapeutic drugs were used in about half of this patient population; antipsychotic drugs were prescribed four times as often as any other psychotherapeutic agent. The popularity of thioridazine was not considered by these authors to be based on firm evidence of its superiority as demonstrated in controlled studies.

A survey conducted by the U.S. Department of Health, Education and Welfare[10] studied patterns of drug usage among a sample of 3,458 residents of 288 long-term care skilled nursing facilities across the United States; the findings provided a picture of the more than 0.25 million such residents in 6,591 skilled nursing homes participating in Medicare/Medicaid programs in 1974, for whom 1,731,360 drug prescriptions were written in that year. The average number of prescriptions per resident was 6.1, but 40% of patients had 7 or more prescriptions, and a few patients received over 20 during the study year.

In this survey, laxatives were the largest single class of drugs prescribed for the largest number of nursing home patients (14.8% of all prescriptions), followed by analgesics (10.8%) and tranquilizers (10.1%). About 60% of patients had prescriptions for laxatives, 51.3% for analgesics, and 46.9% for tranquilizers. The other major groups of drugs used were sedatives/hypnotics and vitamins. Together these five groups comprised nearly half of all prescriptions. It is of interest that in this survey, cardiac drugs accounted for only 5.6% of prescriptions, diuretics 4.1%, antihypertensives 3.4%, antimicrobials 3.1%, vasodilators 2%, and antidepressants a mere 1.5%. The survey was unable to find a pattern in the dosages used for the elderly, in view of the wide variations encountered.

Within the major drug categories, it was found that the commonest drugs employed were:

Laxatives: Magnesium hydroxide, dioctyl sodium sulfosuccinate, danthron, and bisacodyl (together = more than 75% of all laxative prescriptions)

Analgesics: Acetylsalicylic acid (51.3% of all analgesic prescriptions), propoxyphene (31.8%), and acetaminophen (paracetamol) (12.8%)

Tranquilizers: Major (antipsychotics): 64% of all prescriptions for tranquilizers—mainly phenothiazines (thioridazine, 26%, chlorpromazine, 23%).

Minor (antianxiety): mainly benzodiazepines (diazepam, 18%).

The same report compares the patterns found with those in other settings. Analgesics and tranquilizers ranked high in acute hospitals, in the Medicaid program, and in overall national prescribing patterns. Antimicrobials represented a large proportion of prescriptions in all settings *except* nursing homes. The predominant use of laxatives in nursing homes is according to expectation.

A review of laxative use in a skilled nursing facility[51] showed that this class of drugs was used rationally, but that insufficient attention was paid to the dietary management of constipation, particularly the role of a high-fiber diet.

Table 1-4. Fifteen Most Prescribed Therapeutic Classes of Drugs, Belgium, 1981 (ranked according to proportionate use, within each therapeutic class, in subjects aged 65 years or over)

Therapeutic Class	Percent Prescriptions for Patients ≥ 65 Years
Peripheral vasodilators	65.4
Cardiac therapy	56.8
Diuretics	53.5
Ophthalmologicals	32.9
Psycholeptics	32.7
Beta blockers	31.0
Antirheumatics	30.7
Antiasthmatics	29.1
Antiemetics	26.2
Vitamins[a]	22.1
Antispasmodics	20.5
Analgesics[a]	18.0
Cough and cold preparations[a]	14.8
Systemic antibiotics	10.3
Sex hormones	4.8
Additional drugs with major use in the elderly:	
Laxatives[a]	47

[a] Prescribed use reflects only a fraction of total use because of large volume of over-the-counter sales. Data by courtesy of IMS International, Inc.

Table 1-5. Classification of Drugs Included in Tables 1-1–1-4[a]

	Percent Prescriptions for Patients $\geq$ 65 Years			
	U.K.	Germany	Netherlands	Belgium
Analgesics[b]	35	22	(15)	(18)
Narcotic	44	45	31	41
Non-narcotic	36	23	(15)	(17)
Antacids, antiflatulents, and anti–peptic				
ulcer drugs[b]	38	27	44	23
Antacids, antiflatulents	41	30	23	23
Anti–peptic ulcer drugs	29	21	21	21
Others	67	(19)	50	33
Anti-anemics[c]	25	25	17	32
Liver and combinations with vitamin B_{12}	67	24	(15)	23
Iron	23	57	45	44
Others	27	24	25	—
Antiasthmatics	30	41	27	29
Bronchodilators	30	41	27	31
Others	50	56	80	(17)
Antibiotics (systemic)	(13)	(12)	(12)	(10)
Cephalosporins and combinations	(16)	(11)	27	39
Penicillin, streptomycin	—	28	—	38
Rifampicin, rifamycin	100	—	—	59
Carbenicillins	100	24	—	64
Aminoglycosides	53	(7)	—	39
Chloramphenicol	29	24	—	(19)
Antiemetics	41	43	32	26
Antihypertensives	53	64	51	31
Rauwolfia	70	62	(16)	71
Combinations including diuretics	66	66	48	57
Synthetic agents	52	56	61	63
Others	—	73	—	—
Antirheumatics	43	36	25	31
Nonsteroidal	43	38	25	31
Steroidal	43	28	24	26
Antispasmodics	21	24	(17)	21
Beta blockers	42	31	34	31
Alone	43	28	34	31
Combination products	36	37	30	(14)
Cardiac therapy	68	59	60	57
Cardiac and respiratory stimulants	84	22	(19)	28
Glycosides	79	73	78	76
Antianginal	58	60	56	61
Antiarrhythmics	50	55	45	50
Others	79	67	33	44
Cholagogues	42	40	41	32
Corticosteroids (topical)	22	24	(15)	(20)
Alone	22	25	(16)	23
Combination products	21	24	(14)	(16)
Cough and cold preparations[b]	(20)	(18)	(15)	(15)
Antimicrobials	51	—	—	—
Expectorants	33	25	(16)	21
Cough sedatives	(20)	(17)	(16)	(13)
Other	(11)	26	(6)	(4)
Diuretics	59	57	51	54
Nonthiazides	67	59	54	56
Thiazides	55	56	49	51
Laxatives[b]	56	44	41	47
Nasal Decongestants[b]	(8)	(11)	(4)	(7)
Ophthalmologicals	NA	NA	NA	33

Table 1-5. (*continued*)

	Percent Prescriptions for Patients $\geq$ 65 Years			
	U.K.	Germany	Netherlands	Belgium
Peripheral vasodilators	68	67	68	65
Psychoanaleptics	27	40	(19)	31
Neurotropics	80	63	45	69
Neurotonics	33	22	(10)	(18)
Antidepressants	27	33	(19)	(20)
Psycholeptics, antidepressants	27	35	(19)	(17)
Psychostimulants	22	23	(6)	(17)
Psycholeptics	38	41	26	33
Hypnotics, sedatives	50	48	36	43
Neuroleptics	35	32	(20)	26
Tranquilizers	26	37	21	30
Sex hormones	(1)	(3)	(2)	(5)
Vasoprotective drugs	29	42	24	32
Systemic vasoprotectors	44	44	37	35
Topical antivaricose	29	45	34	(19)
Topical antihemorrhoidals	27	32	(17)	26
Vitamins[b]	40	25	29	22
Vitamin B_{12} alone	61	45	61	37
Vitamin C + minerals	49	32	26	(17)
Multivitamins	40	29	35	(10)
Vitamin $B_1 \pm B_6, B_{12}$	39	30	25	27
Vitamin B complex	38	31	25	21
Vitamin A and D combinations	32	(8)	(19)	(20)
Multivitamins + minerals	28	(15)	(19)	(18)

[a] Includes only those with >20% use in the elderly.
[b] Prescribed use reflects only a fraction of total use because of large volume of over-the-counter sales.
[c] For vitamin B_{12}, see vitamins.
Data by courtesy of IMS International, Inc.

Individual smaller studies have added other perspectives to this overall picture.[52-55]

A large study of 5,902 Medicaid patients living in 173 Tennessee nursing homes[56] included a review of 384,326 prescriptions. Of these patients, 43% received antipsychotic drugs during the one-year study period, 9% on a regular daily basis. This figure compares closely with the 46.9% reported in the Department of Health, Education and Welfare survey.[10]

However, Ray et al.[56] consider that this figure represents an excessive use of antipsychotic drugs and adduce evidence to suggest that there is misuse of these drugs in nursing homes, relating to the size of the homes and the patterns of medical care. They conclude that a close examination of this issue is needed and that controlled studies should be carried out in nursing homes to evaluate alternative methods of patient management that rely less on psychotropic drugs. This view echoes the concern of the National Institute on Drug Abuse,[46] cited above.

In a study of a 200-bed long-term-care facility,[57] 61% of the patients were receiving psychotropic drugs. In this study, 46% received diuretics and antihypertensive drugs, 14% cardiotonic agents, and 14% antimicrobials. These figures differ considerably from those of the large Department of Health, Education and Welfare survey described above[10] and are more representative of long-term hospital care.

At the other end of the institutional scale (in homes housing basically fit elderly people), the picture shows other differences. Whereas laxative use remains the commonest medication, there is also widespread use of sedatives/hypnotics and antihypertensive and cardiac drugs, as well as analgesics; but there is less prescription of major tranquilizers (35%) than in skilled nursing facilities.[58]

An analysis of hypnotic usage in 23 residential homes for the elderly in Scotland was reported by Morgan et al.[59] Of a total of 1,122 residents, 34% received hypnotics both on the night of the point-prevalence survey and also on the preceding night. There was wide variability between the homes and no preference for short-half-life hypnotics. The commonest hypnotic used was nitrazepam (33.2% of total usage), a long-acting drug associated with confusional states, cognitive impairment, and residual sedation in elderly persons. Of those receiving this drug, over one quarter received a 10-mg dose, which is now generally regarded as excessive or even contraindicated in this age group.

It is worth remembering that not all long-term facilities have skilled nursing staff. In a survey of a residential home in Scotland, Knox and Melvin[60] found that all but 2 of 35 residents on long-term therapy were incapable of taking responsibility for their own medication. These authors described a system designed to overcome this problem.

This matter was pursued by Bruce,[38] who studied the prescribing of drugs for regular consumption by 20 elderly women in a residential home (with no medical or nursing staff). He considered that only 13 (25%) of the 52 regular prescriptions were justified unequivocally, whereas 20% were no longer necessary. Thirty-eight percent of the prescriptions were for drugs affecting the central nervous system: half of these were stopped without adverse sequelae. Half of the 23% of prescriptions for cardiovascular drugs were also stopped, and only one (a diuretic) had to be reinstituted. The system of Knox and Melvin[60] was used to ensure accuracy of drug administration.

Special attention was paid by Sorensen et al.[61] to the appropriateness of vitamin and mineral prescription orders for elderly residents of four Health Related Facilities in upper New York State. Of 443 subjects, 43 (9.9%) received these preparations inappropriately, and 5 (1.2%) failed to receive a prescription when it would have been medically indicated.

Acute Hospital Experience   The United States pattern of acute hospital prescribing for the elderly has been cited above.[10] A Scottish survey of hospital drug use for the elderly[62] covered one 24-hour period in July, 1975, and included all 873 patients aged 65 and over in all the hospitals in Dundee. Patients in geriatric wards were prescribed most drugs, an average of 4 drugs per patient, as against the overall average of 3.3 drugs per patient, during the 24-hour observation period. Only 15% of the patients received no drugs during that period; 1 patient in 7 received 6 or more drugs per day.

The elderly were prescribed over twice as many p.r.n. (''as required'') drugs as younger patients, which calls to mind pleas[53,63] for more rational use of p.r.n. prescribing. The most widely used drugs were hypnotics (over 400 prescriptions). Chloral derivatives were the most frequently prescribed drugs for patients in geriatric beds, but phenothiazines, diuretics, laxatives, and cardiac drugs were also widely prescribed; elderly patients in medical wards also frequently received mineral supplements and antimicrobials. This type of survey is influenced by p.r.n. prescribing (about half of the patients received such therapy) and by staff/patient ratios.

Among the points made by the authors[62] in their discussion, two are of particular interest in the present context: (1) nitrazepam was prescribed as a hypnotic 96 times; 42 (44%) of these prescriptions were for 10-mg doses despite the fact that the official data sheet for this drug recommends up to 5 mg for elderly patients; (2) amitriptyline, given once daily, late in the evening, could provide effective antidepressant therapy and at the same time eliminate the need for night sedation. Yet tricyclics were often prescribed two or three times a day.

The authors concluded that there was excessive use of hypnotics, and little dose reduction was noted with increasing age. They called for further evaluation of hospital drug prescribing for the elderly, with a view to more appropriate modifications that could lead to improved response and fewer adverse effects.

Salzman and van der Kolk[64] surveyed drug prescriptions for the elderly (60 years and over) in a general hospital in Boston on a single weekday in 1978. The study included 348 patients of all ages; 142 (41%) received a psychotropic drug on the survey day, and of this number, 44% were aged 60 or over. Of the total of 195 patients in the study aged 60 and over, 62 (32%) received a psychotropic drug. The commonest psychoactive agents used were hypnotics (nearly 75% of the elderly patients), especially flurazepam. In this study, 23% of the elderly received sedative/hypnotic drugs for indications other than sleep. In the Boston Collaborative Drug Survey,[65] flurazepam was used by 43% of patients aged over 60; rather large doses (30 mg) predominated.

Of the remaining psychoactive drugs in the Salzman and van der Kolk study,[64] antianxiety drugs were used in 35% of the elderly patients; diazepam (average dose 15 mg daily) was used almost exclusively. No patients received neuroleptic drugs for psychotic symptoms. Salzman and van der Kolk[64] comment that the benzodiazepine dosages noted in their survey were probably too high. The few patients on antidepressants had been taking them before admission to the hospital.

SELF-MEDICATION AND COMPLIANCE

Self-medication is common in the elderly, but a far greater degree of education is needed.[66] Self-medication of prescribed drugs is of particular concern when patients are discharged home from institutions.[30] In hospitals and extended care facilities, drugs are usually given by a nurse up to the point of discharge, without efforts being made to ensure that the patient is capable of adhering to the recommended requirements—which may at times be quite complex. Libow and Mehl[67] demonstrated the value of educating long-term hospital inpatients to administer their own drugs over a two-week period.

It is well known that elderly chronically ill outpatients make many medication errors,[68] and attempts have been made by some geriatricians to teach selected patients to administer their own drugs, under appropriate supervision, prior to discharge from hospitals. Clearly, there are many practical difficulties in carrying out such a program, but it would seem to be a worthwhile endeavor.[69,70] If such a scheme is not possible, it is still of value to spend some time on personal instruction of patients regarding drugs (and also diet, exercise, physical therapy, and so on, as appropriate) prior to discharge from hospitals.[2,71]

Without such special attention, whether in a hospital or the doctor's office, a substantial proportion of elderly patients fail to comply with accurate self-medication because of lack of understanding,[72,73] and this cause of noncompliance is commoner than other (admittedly important) factors, such as visual or mental deterioration. For further discussion of compliance in the elderly, see references 2, 21 and 74–76.

Self-medication with OTC drugs is discussed elsewhere in this volume. It may be pointed out here, however, that the use of nonprescribed drugs can lead to interactions with prescribed medications, or to adverse reactions due to the OTC drug itself.[77]

MISUSE AND ABUSE OF DRUGS BY THE ELDERLY: ADVERSE DRUG REACTIONS

Much misuse of drugs by the elderly remains unknown unless it produces some kind of problem or crisis.[43] Nearly one in five patients admitted to the geriatric department of a general hospital had symptoms attributable to the effects of prescribed drugs.[78,79] This incidence resembles the 15.4% reported by Hurwitz[14] for adverse drug reactions in the elderly (aged 60 or over) admitted to a general hospital. The experience reported from a multicenter British study of geriatric departments[80] was somewhat less (12.5%). Psychogeriatric hospital experience in Australia[81] showed that at least 16% of 236 admissions had adverse effects from psychotropic drugs at the time of admission, and these patients improved rapidly when the offending drugs were withdrawn. Further, it was estimated that "at least 20% of admissions to a psychogeriatric unit are directly due to medication."[81]

Caranasos et al.[82] found that 177 (2.9%) of 6,063 consecutive admissions to a general hospital were due to adverse drug effects; of these 177 patients, 41% were aged over 60 years, and there was a modest increase in the incidence of adverse drug effects from 60 to 80 years compared with younger ages.[12]

Alcoholism in the elderly is discussed later in this chapter.

DRUG INTERACTIONS IN THE ELDERLY

Several recent accounts give examples of drug interactions that are of particular relevance in the elderly,[11,77,83,84] including reactions between drugs and food and nutritional status.[85,86] Of particular value is the contribution of Blaschke et al.,[11] who reported data on prescribing habits and the frequency of potential drug/drug interactions in a series of nursing homes in the eastern United States. They made use of a computer-based system[87] and showed that psychotropic drugs and anticoagulants were most frequently involved in drug interactions. It is also significant that, whereas 20% of *patients* received a potentially interacting combination, only 7% of *prescriptions* were considered potentially interacting.

SOME SPECIFIC DRUG GROUPS

Cardiac Glycosides

In any account of drug use in the elderly, specific mention of cardiac glycosides is mandatory. Digoxin is the seventh most frequently prescribed drug in the United States.[88] Digitalis preparations are frequently prescribed for elderly patients and are often continued over prolonged periods without clear evidence as to their continuing benefit[31] or the appropriateness of the maintenance dosage.[32,33,89] In the United Kingdom, nearly 80% of patients receiving digoxin are over 60 years of age; 60% are over 70 years old.[90,91] It has been estimated that 5%–6% of the entire population over 65 in the United Kingdom take digoxin.[90,92] In Sweden, 14%–18% of the population in their eighth decade receive a cardiac glycoside.[93] These drugs have a narrow therapeutic ratio, and digoxin toxicity increases sharply after the age of 60 years.[91] The toxicity is not due to increased sensitivity of the aging body to digoxin, but to reduced renal function in the elderly. The half-life of digoxin increases by over one third in the elderly with reduced creatinine clearance.* Digitoxin is metabolized differently from digoxin, undergoing extensive biotransformation in the liver, but its half-life is over one week, compared with 1.8 days for digoxin.

Diuretics

There is overuse of diuretics in the elderly, particularly with long-term administration.[35,36] Most diuretics increase potassium loss; the loss may be minimized by using low doses, but the elderly have low potassium reserves and frequently have suboptimal dietary intakes of potassium[94] so that even low-dose diuretics may induce potassium deficiency. Attention should be paid to dietary potassium in the elderly, especially those on diuretics.

The use of oral potassium supplements in the elderly carries with it many problems: combinations of diuretics and potassium are not recommended, usually providing too little potassium and sometimes causing gastrointestinal adverse effects; large doses of potassium chloride may be needed, and will almost always present difficulties in compliance.

---

* Note that creatinine clearance may be much reduced in the presence of normal serum creatinine and urea.

Judicious use of a potassium-sparing diuretic in combination with a thiazide may be of value to prevent hypokalemia in the elderly, provided renal function is known to be adequate.

Beta Blockers

Age-related pharmacokinetic[95,96] and pharmacodynamic[97] changes have been described for beta blockers. These drugs are not always easy to use in the elderly[22] and are sometimes given inappropriately. They are especially popular in the United Kingdom and Sweden.

Antihypertensive Drugs

Antihypertensive drugs require great caution in selection and use in the elderly—as does the selection of patients to receive them. The subject is too vast to consider in detail here; the reader is referred to reviews.[98-104] The situation may be summarized thus: Severe hypertension requires treatment at any age. Mild to moderate hypertension in the elderly is associated with increased morbidity and mortality,[105] but the benefits of therapy in this age group remain controversial. Reports of studies being carried out under the aegis of the European Working Party on Hypertension in the Elderly and the Medical Research Council (United Kingdom) are awaited.

Anticoagulants

The elderly may show increased sensitivity to heparin[106] and to warfarin.[107,108] The elderly may be relatively deficient in vitamin K because of decreased intake and/or absorption, or because of pharmacokinetic changes.[108,109]

Analgesics

The widespread use of analgesics by the elderly has been described above; this usage includes OTC drugs as well as prescription drugs.[77]

Propoxyphene has had a frequent usage but has lost popularity in the United States because of reports that dependence may occur; interactions with alcohol may be serious and have sometimes been fatal. Doubt has also been cast on the degree of efficacy when combined with another analgesic, such as acetylsalicylic acid or acetaminophen (paracetamol).

Sedative/Hypnotic and Anxiolytic Agents

Barbiturates are now generally accepted as having little place in treating the elderly. Chloral is still widely used; though somewhat old-fashioned, it is safe and predictable in its effect. Enzyme induction may occur, but to a lesser extent than at younger ages.[110]

Benzodiazepines have been the subject of much valuable research in recent years, particularly in regard to their usage in the elderly. There have been reports of an increased incidence of unwanted sedation with increasing age from chlordiazepoxide and diazepam,[111] nitrazepam,[112] and flurazepam.[65] The findings for nitrazepam were confirmed and extended by Castleden et al.,[113] who showed increased receptor sensitivity to this drug in their elderly subjects.

Short-acting benzodiazepines (oxazepam, tamezepam, or lorazepam) are preferable in the elderly. Nevertheless, widespread use of the long-acting agents persists, and, as noted previously in this chapter, the doses prescribed are often too large for elderly subjects. If flurazepam is used in the elderly, the hypnotic dose should not exceed 15 mg; for nitrazepam, the initial dose should be only 2.5 mg, increasing to 5 mg after one week if necessary. Intermittent therapy is best for benzodiazepines since some degree of dependence is possible.

Chlormethiazole has shown increasing popularity as a hypnotic for geriatric patients in the United Kingdom and other parts of Europe,[114,115] but pharmacokinetic changes mean that reduced dosage is often required.[116]

Antidepressants

Tricyclics (and ***tetracyclics***) are probably used less often in the elderly than might be warranted; but it is important to begin with low doses to establish safety, since adverse effects are common in old age because of age-related pharmacokinetic and pharmacodynamic changes.[12]

Monoamine oxidase inhibitors are not easy to administer in the elderly because of the dietary restrictions required, the possibility of drug interactions, and other adverse effects. They are rarely used in this age group.

Lithium usage calls for careful biochemical control.

Stimulants have little place in the elderly.

Newer antidepressants, such as nomifensine and viloxazine, are coming into use more frequently in the elderly; these drugs—especially nomifensine—are claimed to be better tolerated than tricyclics. Zimelidine may be even better for the elderly.

Neuroleptics (Antipsychotic Drugs)

Phenothiazines are the most frequently prescribed drugs in this category, especially thioridazine and chlorpromazine. Side effects are more common in the elderly than at younger ages.[117]

Butyrophenones (e.g., haloperidol) are used for sedation and to help reduce hallucinations.

Antiparkinsonism Drugs

Anticholinergic and antihistamine drugs are still used, but may produce confusion and hallucinations. Levodopa revolutionized the treatment of parkinsonism but was difficult to use in the elderly prior to the introduction of dopa decarboxylase inhibitors. Now, Sinemet (MSD) or Madopar (Roche) allow much benefit to be realized by the elderly.

Cerebroactive Drugs

The term *cerebroactive drugs*[118,119] embraces cerebral vasodilators, metabolic improvers, and similar agents used in attempts to improve brain function in elderly patients with dementia. This area is controversial, though highly important; unfortunately there are insufficient hard data for adequate evaluation of this heterogeneous group of drugs. Nevertheless, they are widely used for the elderly in parts of Europe.

Alcohol

Alcohol, taken with other drugs, accounts for a considerable amount of abuse after age 50.[120] A Gallup poll[121] indicated that the elderly shared in the rising trend toward alcohol consumption in the population as a whole; 54% of those over 50 were users of alcohol. Gerbino[122] gives an even higher figure (61%). Moss and Beresford-Davies[123] reported that 9% of the alcoholics they found in a community survey in Cambridgeshire, England, were over 65 years old. In Geneva, Switzerland, 10% of alcoholics were over 60 years old in the study of Favre and de Meuron.[124] Cisin and Cahalan[125] reported that 6% of subjects over 60 in a national survey in the United States were heavy drinkers. Bailey et al.[126] noted that, in New York City, 2.2% of their study population aged 65–74 and 1.2% of those over 75 years old had drinking problems. Zimberg,[127] also in New York, reported that of 87 patients aged 65 and over admitted to a suburban community mental health center, 17% had a drinking problem.

Guttman[43] surveyed 447 persons aged 60 and over living in the community in Washington, D.C. The majority (56.2%) reported little or no use of alcohol; 24.6% drank "infrequently," and 18.6% "frequently." Only 3.3% used spirits, and only 1.1% said that problems resulted from the use of alcohol.

It is difficult to compare all these studies, with different populations and different methods, but it is probable that many elderly alcoholics remain undiagnosed and untreated.[128-130] Brody[131] pointed out that surveys were expensive ways to obtain potentially inaccurate information on alcoholism and called for a major preventive and education program in middle age.

Glatt et al.[132] reported on studies in London involving 195 elderly patients referred to a geriatric unit (36 patients) or an alcoholism unit (159 patients). They noted a preponderance of women over men and a relative excess of widows compared to widowers. Personality factors were much less important among older alcoholics than among younger alcoholics. Social or psychosocial factors, possibly complicated by disease, were important in those patients (just over half) who were not long-standing heavy drinkers. In his community survey, Guttman[43] reported that 80% of the subjects gave social and psychological reasons for using alcohol, but only 30% related this to a personal problem.

Glatt et al.[132] discuss briefly the detection, management, and prevention of alcoholism in the elderly, stressing, among other things, attention to regular food intake to prevent the substitution of drink for food by some old people.

Interactions between alcohol and drug therapy in the elderly have been discussed in detail by several authors,[122,133,134] who emphasize the importance of increased awareness by physicians of this possibility.

Antidiabetic Drugs

Oral hypoglycemic agents are frequently prescribed for elderly diabetic patients. They should not be used when diet alone can control the problem. When they are indicated, care should be taken to avoid chlorpropamide, since its half-life approaches 36 hours and may be prolonged further by interaction with other drugs. In addition, chlorpropamide potentiates vasopressin and may lead to dilutional hyponatremia, which is poorly tolerated by the elderly. Biguanides are also best avoided because of the risk of lactic acidosis and nonketotic hyperosmolar diabetic coma, seen particularly in the elderly. Complications of drug treatment of elderly diabetics are discussed by Rifkin.[135]

Nonsteroidal Anti-Inflammatory Drugs (NSAIDs)

During 1981, 6 million (30%) of the prescriptions for NSAIDs in the United Kingdom were for elderly patients with osteoarthritis. Concomitant use of a NSAID to help control inflammation and an analgesic to relieve any residual pain has been advocated as being probably the therapy of choice in many elderly arthritics.[136]

Whereas NSAIDs have proved of considerable value for the elderly with rheumatic disorders (mainly osteoarthritis and rheumatoid arthritis) when control of inflammation is required, there is an increased incidence of adverse effects attending the use of NSAIDs in the elderly—especially gastrointestinal bleeding and symptomless ulceration[137] and also occasional deterioration of renal function.[138] Although there is little choice between most of the NSAIDs in this respect, there is growing evidence that one NSAID, sulindac, is less likely than the others to produce these symptoms; this drug is absorbed in an inactive (prodrug) form, which may produce less gastrointestinal disturbances, and sulindac appears not to inhibit the synthesis of renal prostaglandins.[139,140] It has been suggested that older patients would benefit from a NSAID that did not inhibit renal prostaglandins.[141]

SUMMARY

The growing numbers of the elderly and the multiple pathology that affects them inevitably lead to increased use of drugs in old age. This use carries the risks of overprescribing (inappropriate or excessive drug use [diuretics, digoxin, psychoactive drugs, iron]; excessive dosage [digoxin, benzodiazepines]; and overlong drug use [diuretics, digoxin]), which may be complicated by OTC drug use. The incidence of adverse reactions with age, and drug interactions are more likely in the elderly.

Patterns of prescribing for the elderly are examined in the community and in institutions, with examples from the United States and Europe. Drugs affecting the central nervous system and the cardiovascular system are undoubtedly those in commonest use, although laxatives are, not surprisingly, extensively used in institutions. Interesting differences in international practice include the popularity of peripheral vasodilators in Germany and Belgium, beta blockers in the United Kingdom, and topical antirheumatics in Germany.

There is need for greater education regarding self-medication, which would help increase compliance and reduce errors.

Various drug groups are considered briefly with regard to their use in the elderly; alcohol is included, as alcoholism often goes unrecognized in old age.

ACKNOWLEDGMENTS

The author acknowledges with thanks the assistance of Tom Oberleiton of Marketing Research, Merck Sharp & Dohme International, and those colleagues in the Department of Medical and Scientific Affairs, Merck Sharp & Dohme International , who have helped in the preparation of this chapter; also IMS International, Inc., for the data used in Tables 1–5.

REFERENCES

1. Gershon S, Herman SP: The differential diagnosis of dementia. J Am Geriat Soc 30 (suppl): S58–S66, 1982.
2. World Health Organization: Health care in the elderly: Report of the Technical Group on the Use of Medicaments by the Elderly. Drugs 22:279–294, 1981.
3. Gibson RM, Mueller M, Fisher CR: Age differences in health care spending. Fiscal year 1976. Soc Sec Bull 40:3–14, 1977.
4. O'Malley K, Judge TG, Crooks J: Geriatric clinical pharmacology and therapeutics. In Avery GS (ed): Drug Treatment. Edinburgh, Churchill Livingstone, 1976, pp 123–142.
5. Neugarten BL, Havighurst RJ: Aging and the future. In Neugarten BL, Havighurst RJ (eds): Social Policy, Social Ethics, and the Aging Society. Washington, DC, United States Government Printing Office, 1976.
6. Law R, Chalmers C: Medicine and elderly people: A general practice survey. Br Med J 1:565–568, 1976.
7. Shaw SM, Opit LJ: Need for supervision in the elderly receiving long-term prescribed medication. Br Med J 1:503–507, 1976.
8. Achong MR, Bayne JRD, Gerson LW, Golshani S: Prescribing of psychoactive drugs for chronically ill elderly patients. Can Med Assoc J 118:1503–1508, 1978.
9. Cape R: Aging: Its Complex Management. Hagerstown, Md, Harper & Row, 1978.
10. United States Department of Health, Education and Welfare: Physicians' Drug Prescribing Patterns in Skilled Nursing Facilities. Long-Term Care Facility Improvement

Campaign. Monograph No 2. Washington, DHEW, Office of Long-Term Care, 1976.

11. Blaschke TF, Cohen SN, Tatro DS, Rubin PC: Drug-drug interactions and aging. In Jarvik LF, Greenblatt DJ, Harman D (eds): Clinical Pharmacology and the Aged Patient. New York, Raven Press, 1981, pp 11–26.

12. O'Malley K, Laher M, Cusack B, Kelly JG: Clinial pharmacology and the elderly patient. In Denham MJ (ed): The Treatment of Medical Problems in the Elderly. Lancaster, England, MTP Press Ltd, 1980, pp 1–33.

13. Seidl LG, Thorton GF, Smith JW, Cluff LF: Studies on the epidemiology of adverse drug reactions. Bull Johns Hopkins Hosp 119:299–315, 1966.

14. Hurwitz N: Predisposing factors in adverse reactions to drugs. Br Med J 1:536–539, 1969.

15. Klein U, Klein M, Stern H, Rothenbühler M, et al: The frequency of adverse drug reactions as dependent upon age, sex and duration of hospitalization. Int J Clin Pharmacol Biopharm 13:187–195, 1976.

16. May FE, Stewart RB, Cluff LE: Drug interaction and multiple drug administration. Clin Pharmacol Ther 22:322–328, 1977.

17. Lawson DH, Jick H: Drug prescribing in hospitals: An international comparison. Am J Publ Hlth 66:644–648, 1976.

18. Triggs EJ, Nation RL: Pharmacokinetics in the aged: A review. J Pharmacokin Biopharm 3:387–418, 1975.

19. Crooks J, O'Malley K, Stevenson IH: Pharmacokinetics in the elderly. Clin Pharmacokin 1:280–296, 1976.

20. Richey DP, Bender AD: Pharmacokinetic consequences of aging. Ann Rev Pharmacol Toxicol 17:49–65, 1977.

21. Vestal RE: Drug use in the elderly: A review of problems and special considerations. Drugs 16:358–382, 1978.

22. Vestal RE: Pharmacology and aging. J Am Geriat Soc 30:191–200, 1982.

23. Greenblatt DJ, Divoll M, Abernethy DR, Shader RI: Physiologic changes in old age. Relation to altered drug disposition. J Am Geriat Soc 30 (suppl):S6–S10, 1982.

24. Scott PJW: Review: The effect of age on pharmacodynamics in man. J Clin Exp Gerontol 4:205–226, 1982.

25. Crombie DL, Green CM, Pearce AJ, et al: Supervision of repeat prescribing. Br Med J 1:713, 1976.

26. Forbes JA; Prescribing for the elderly in general practice and the problems of record keeping. Geront Clin 16:14–17, 1974.

27. Manasse AP: Repeat prescriptions in general practice. J Roy Coll Gen Pract 24:203–207, 1974.

28. Dawson PJ: Consultations and treatment in the elderly. Practitioner 224:466–467, 1980.

29. Tulloch AJ: Repeat prescribing for elderly patients. Br Med J 282:1672–1675, 1981.

30. Gibson IIJM, O'Hare MM: Prescription of drugs for older people at home. Geront Clin 10:271–280, 1968.

31. Dall JLC: Maintenance digoxin in elderly patients. Br Med J 2:705–706, 1970.

32. Hull S, Mackintosh A: Discontinuation of maintenance digoxin therapy in general practice. Lancet 2:1054–1055, 1977.

33. Johnston GD, McDevitt DG: Is maintenance digoxin necessary in patients with sinus rhythm? Lancet 1:567–570, 1979.

34. Fleg JL, Gottlieb SH, Lakatta EG: Is digoxin really important in treatment of compensated heart failure? A placebo-controlled crossover study in patients with sinus rhythm. Am J Med 73:244–250, 1982.

35. Burr ML, King S, Davies HEF, Pathy MS: The effects of discontinuing long-term diuretic therapy in the elderly. Age and Ageing 6:38–45, 1977.
36. Myers MG, Weingert ME, Fisher RH, et al: Unnecessary diuretic therapy in the elderly. Age and Ageing 11:213–221, 1982.
37. Reizenstein P, Ljunggren G, Smcdby B, et al: Overprescribing iron tablets to elderly people in Sweden. Br Med J 2:962–963, 1979.
38. Bruce SA: Regular prescribing in a residential home for elderly women. Br Med J 284:1235–1237, 1982.
39. Kohn R, White KL: Health Care: An International Study. London, Oxford University Press, 1976.
40. Boethius G: Recording of drug prescriptions in the county of Jämtland, Sweden. Pattern of drug usage in 16,600 individuals during 1970-75. Acta Med Scand 202:241–251, 1977.
41. Task Force on Prescription Drugs: United States Department of Health, Education and Welfare. Washington, DC, Office of the Secretary, 1968.
42. Chien CP, Townsend EJ, Townsend A: Substance use and abuse among the community elderly: The medical aspect. Addic Dis 3:357–372, 1978.
43. Guttman D: Patterns of legal drug use by older Americans. Addic Dis 3:337–356, 1978.
44. Freeman GK: Drug-prescribing patterns in the elderly: A general practice study. In Crooks J, Stevenson IH (eds): Drugs and the Elderly: Perspectives in Geriatric Clinical Pharmacology. London, Macmillan; Baltimore, University Park Press, 1979, pp 223–229.
45. Stewart RB, Hale WE, Marks RG: Analgesic drug use in an ambulatory elderly population. Drug Intell Clin Pharm 16:833–836, 1982.
46. NIDA: The Aging Process and Psychoactive Drug Use. National Institute on Drug Abuse Services Research Monograph Series. Publ. No 79-813. Washington, United States Government Printing Office; Menlo Park, Ca, Stanford Research Institute, 1979.
47. Knox JDE: Prescribing for the elderly in general practice: A review of current literature. J Roy Coll Gen Pract 30 (suppl 1):1–8, 1980.
48. Skegg DCG, Doll R, Perry J: Use of medicines in general practice. Br Med J 1:1561–1563, 1977.
49. May FE, Stewart RB, Hale WE, Marks RG: Prescribed and nonprescribed drug use in an ambulatory elderly population. South Med J 75:522–528, 1982.
50. Prien RF, Caffey EM Jr: Pharmacologic treatment of elderly patients with organic brain syndrome: A survey of twelve Veterans' Administration Hospitals. Comp Psych 18:551–560, 1977.
51. Lamy PP, Krug BH: Review of laxative utilization in a skilled nursing facility. J Am Geriat Soc 26:544–549, 1978.
52. Ingman SR, Lawson IR, Pierpaoli PG, Blake P: A survey of the prescribing and administration of drugs in a long-term care institution for the elderly. J Am Geriat Soc 23:309–316, 1975.
53. Howard JB, Strong KE Sr, Strong KE Jr: Medication procedures in a nursing home: Abuse of prn orders. J Am Geriat Soc 25:83–84, 1977.
54. Cooper JW Jr, Bagwell CG: Contribution of the consultant pharmacist to rational drug usage in the long-term care facility. J Am Geriat Soc 26:513–520, 1978.
55. Segal JR, Thompson JF, Floyd RA: Drug utilization and prescribing patterns in a skilled nursing facility: The need for a rational approach to therapeutics. J Am Geriat Soc 27:117–122, 1979.
56. Ray WA, Federspiel CF, Schaffner W: A study of antipsychotic drug use in nursing homes: Epidemiologic evidence suggesting misuse. Am J Publ Hlth 70:485–491, 1980.

57. Kalchthaler T, Coccaro E, Lichtiger S: Incidence of polypharmacy in a long-term care facility. J Am Geriat Soc 25:308–313, 1977.
58. Lyle WM: Drugs prescribed for the elderly. J Am Optometric Assoc 48:1029–1032, 1977.
59. Morgan K, Gilleard CJ, Reive A: Hypnotic usage in residential homes for the elderly: A prevalence and longitudinal analysis. Age and Ageing 11:229–234, 1982.
60. Knox JDE, Melvin M: Prescribed medicines in a residential home for the elderly. Nursing Times 76:1934–1936, 1980.
61. Sorensen AA, Sorensen DI, Zimmer JG: Appropriateness of vitamin and mineral prescription orders for residents of Health Related Facilities. J Am Geriat Soc 27:425–430, 1979.
62. Christopher LJ, Ballinger BR, Shepherd AMM, et al: A survey of hospital prescribing for the elderly. In Crooks J, Stevenson IH (eds): Drugs and the Elderly: Perspectives in Geriatric Clinical Pharmacology. London, Macmillan; Baltimore, University Park Press, 1979, pp 231–238.
63. Howard JB, Strong KE Sr, Strong KE Jr: Nursing home medication costs. J Am Geriat Soc 26:228–230, 1978.
64. Salzman C, Van Der Kolk B: Psychotropic drug prescriptions for elderly patients in a general hospital. J Am Geriat Soc 28:18–22, 1980.
65. Greenblatt DJ, Allen MD, Shader RI: Toxicity of high-dose flurazepam in the elderly. Clin Pharmacol Ther 21:355–361, 1977.
66. Adamson KA, Smith DL: Nonprescription drugs and the elderly patient. Can Pharm J 4:80–85, 1978.
67. Libow LS, Mehl B: Self-administration of medications by patients in hospitals or extended care facilities. J Am Geriat Soc 18:81–85, 1970.
68. Schwartz D, Wang M, Qeitz L, Goss MEW: Medication errors made by elderly, chronically ill patients. Am J Publ Hlth 52:2018–2029, 1962.
69. Wandless I, Davie KW: Can drug compliance in the elderly be improved? Br Med J 1:359–361, 1977.
70. Atkinson L, Gibson I, Andrews J: An investigation into the ability of elderly patients continuing to take drugs after discharge from hospital and recommendations concerning improving the situation. Gerontology 24:225–234, 1978.
71. MacDonald ET, MacDonald JB, Phoenix M: Improving drug compliance after hospital discharge. Br Med J 2:618–621, 1977.
72. Gibson IIJM: Hospital drugs in the home. Geront Clin 16:10–13, 1974.
73. Parkin DM, Henney CR, Quirk J, Crooks J: Deviation from prescribed drug treatment after discharge from hospital. Br Med J 2:686–688, 1976.
74. Wade OL: Compliance problems. In Crooks J, Stevenson IH (eds): Drugs and the Elderly: Perspectives in Geriatric Pharmacology. London, Macmillan; Baltimore, University Park Press, 1979, pp 287–291.
75. Fedder DO: Managing medications and compliance: Physician-pharmacist-patient interactions. J Am Geriat Soc 30 (suppl): S113–S117, 1982.
76. Reinken J, Sparrow M, Campbell AJ: The giving and taking of psychotropic drugs in New Zealand. NZ Med J 95:489–492, 1982.
77. Lamy PP: Over-the-counter medication: The drug interactions we overlook. J Am Geriat Soc 30 (suppl): S69–S75, 1982.
78. Wynne RD, Heller F: Drug overuse among the elderly: A growing problem. Perspectives on Aging 11:15–18, 1973.
79. Pascarelli EF: Drug dependence: An age-old problem compounded by old age. Geriatrics 29:109–115, 1974.

80. Williamson J, Chopin JM: Adverse reactions to prescribed drugs in the elderly: A multicentre investigation. Age and Ageing 9:73–80, 1980.
81. Learoyd BM: Psychotropic drugs and the elderly patient. Mcd J Aust 1:1131–1133, 1972.
82. Caranasos GJ, Stewart RB, Cluff E: Drug-induced illness leading to hospitalization. JAMA 228:713–717, 1974.
83. Hyams DE: Drugs in the elderly: Uses, abuses and interactions. In Andrews J, Von Hahn HP (eds): Geriatrics for Everyday Practice, Basel, Karger, 1981, pp 193–212.
84. Reidenberg MM: Drug interactions and the elderly. J Am Geriat Soc 30 (suppl): S67–S68, 1982.
85. Lamy PP: Prescribing for the elderly. Littleton, Mass, PSG Publishing, 1980.
86. Lamy PP: Effects of diet and nutrition on drug therapy. J Am Geriat Soc 30 (suppl): S99–S112, 1982.
87. Cohen SN, Armstrong MF, Briggs RL, et al: A computer-based system for the study and control of drug interactions in hospitalized patients. In Morselli PL, Garattini S, Cohen SN (eds): Drug Interactions, New York, Raven Press, 1974, pp 363–374.
88. Stults BM: Digoxin use in the elderly. J Am Geriat Soc 30:158–164, 1982.
89. Whiting B, Wandless I, Sumner DJ, Goldberg A: A computer-assisted review of digoxin therapy in the elderly. Br Heart J 40:8–13, 1978.
90. Pedoe HDT: Digoxin prescribing in general practice 1967–1977. Lancet 2:931–933, 1978.
91. Whiting B, Lawrence JR, Sumner DJ: Digoxin pharmacokinetics in the elderly. In Crooks J, Stevenson IH (eds): Drugs and the Elderly: Perspectives in Geriatric Clinical Pharmacology. London, Macmillan; Baltimore, University Park Press, 1979, pp 89–101.
92. Taylor BB, Kennedy RD, Caird FI: Digoxin studies in the elderly. Age and Ageing 3:79–84, 1974.
93. Landahl S, Lindblad B, Roupe B, Steen B, Svanborg A: Digitalis therapy in a 70-year-old population. Acta Med Scand 202:437–443, 1977.
94. Judge TG: Potassium and magnesium. In Exton-Smith AN, Caird FI (eds): Metabolic and Nutritional Disorders in the Elderly. Bristol, John Wright and Sons Ltd, 1980, pp 39–44.
95. Castleden CM, Kaye CM, Parsons RL: The effect of age on plasma levels of propranolol and practolol in man. Br J Clin Pharmacol 2:303–306, 1975.
96. Castleden CM, George CF: The effect of ageing on the hepatic clearance of propranolol. Br J Clin Pharmacol 7:49–54, 1979.
97. Vestal RE, Wood AJJ, Shand DG: Reduced beta-adrenoceptor sensitivity in the elderly. Clin Pharmacol Ther 26:181–186, 1979.
98. Koch-Weser J: Treatment of hypertension in the elderly. In Crooks J, Stevenson IH (eds): Drugs and the Elderly: Perspectives in Clinical Pharmacology. London, Macmillan; Baltimore, University Park Press, 1979, pp 247–262.
99. Kirkendall WM, Hammond JJ: Hypertension in the elderly: Arch Intern Med 140:1155–1161, 1980.
100. Niarchos AP, Laragh JH: Hypertension in the elderly: 1. Pathophysiology. Mod Concepts Cardiovasc Dis 49:43–48, 1980.
101. Niarchos AP, Laragh JH: Hypertension in the elderly: 2. Diagnosis and treatment. Mod Concepts Cardiovasc Dis 49:49–54, 1980.
102. O'Malley K, O'Brien E: Management of hypertension in the elderly. New Engl J Med 302:1397–1401, 1980.
103. Libow LS, Butler RN: Treating mild diastolic hypertension in the elderly: Uncertain benefits and possible dangers. Geriatrics 36(11):55–64, 1981.

104. Radin AM, Black HR: Hypertension in the elderly: The time has come to treat. J Am Geriat Soc 29:193–200, 1981.
105. Kannel WB, Gordon T: Evaluation of cardiovascular risk in the elderly: The Framingham Study. Bull NY Acad Med 54:573–591, 1978.
106. Jick H, Slone D, Borda IT, Shapiro S: Efficacy and toxicity of heparin in relation to age and sex. New Engl J Med 279:284–286, 1968.
107. O'Malley K, Stevenson IH, Ward CA, et al: Determinants of anticoagulant control in patients receiving warfarin. Br J Clin Pharmacol 4:309–314, 1977.
108. Shepherd AMM, Hewick DS, Moreland TA, Stevenson IH: Age as a determinant of sensitivity to warfarin. Br J Clin Pharmacol 4:315–320, 1977.
109. Shepherd AMM, Wilson N, Stevenson IH: Warfarin sensitivity in the elderly. In Crooks J, Stevenson IH (eds): Drugs and the Elderly: Perspectives in Clinical Pharmacology. London, Macmillan; Baltimore, University Park Press, 1979, pp 199–209.
110. Salem SAM, Rajjayabun P, Shepherd AMM, Stevenson IH: Reduced induction of drug metabolism in the elderly. Age and Ageing, 7:68–73, 1978.
111. Boston Collaborative Drug Surveillance Program: Clinical depression of the central nervous system due to diazepam and chlordiazepoxide in relation to cigarette smoking and age. New Engl J Med 228:277–280, 1973.
112. Greenblatt DJ, Allen MD: Toxicity of nitrazepam in the elderly: A report from the Boston Collaborative Drug Surveillance Program. Br J Clin Pharmacol 5:407–413, 1978.
113. Castleden CM, George CF, Marcer D, Hallett C: Increased sensitivity to nitrazepam in old age. Br Med J 1:10–12, 1977.
114. Pathy MS: Comparison of two sedative hypnotic drugs. Age and Ageing 6(suppl):91–94, 1977.
115. Nayal S, Castleden CM, George CF, Marcer D: The effect of an hypnotic with a short half-life on hangover effect in old patients. Age and Ageing 7 (suppl):50–54, 1978.
116. Triggs EJ: Pharmacokinetics of lignocaine and chlormethiazole in the elderly; Drugs & the Elderly: with some preliminary observations on other drugs. In Crooks J, Stevenson IH (eds): Perspectives in Clinical Pharmacology. London, Macmillan; Baltimore, University Park Press, 1979, pp 117–132.
117. Salzman C, Shader RI, Van Der Kolk BA: Clinical psychopharmacology and the elderly patient. NY State J Med 76:71–77, 1976.
118. Hyams DE: Cerebral function and drug therapy: The use of cerebral vasodilators, "vasorelaxants," "haemokinators," and "activators." In Brocklehurst JC (ed): Textbook of Geriatric Medicine and Gerontology, 2nd ed. Edinburgh and London, Churchill Livingstone, 1978, pp 670–711.
119. Hyams DE: Cerebral activating drugs. In Denham MJ (ed): The Treatment of Medical Problems in the Elderly. Lancaster, England, MTP Press Ltd, 1980, pp 295–331.
120. Pascarelli EF, Fischer W: Drug dependence in the elderly. Int J Aging Hum Dev 5:347–356, 1974.
121. Gallup G: The rising number of drinkers. Washington Post, June 10, 1974.
122. Gerbino PP: Complications of alcohol use combined with drug therapy in the elderly. J Am Geriat Soc 30 (suppl): S88–S93, 1982.
123. Moss MC, Beresford-Davies E: A survey of alcoholism in an English County: A study of prevalence distribution and effects of alcoholism in Cambridgeshire. UK, Geigy, 1967.
124. Favre A, De Meuron B: Aspect psychosocial de l'alcoolisme de l'âge. Praxis 52:711–716, 1963.

125. Cisin IH, Cahalan D: Comparison of abstainers and heavy drinkers in a national survey. In Cole J (ed): Clinical Research in Alcoholism. Psychiatric Research Report No. 24, American Psychiatric Association, 1968, pp 10–22.
126. Bailey MB, Haberman PW, Alksne H: The epidemiology of alcoholism in an urban residential area. Q J Stud Alc 26:19–40, 1965.
127. Zimberg S: The elderly alcoholic. Gerontologist 14:221–224, 1974.
128. Droller H: Some aspects of alcoholism in the elderly. Lancet 2:137–139, 1964.
129. Rosin AJ, Glatt MM: Alcohol excess in the elderly. Q J Stud Alc 32:53–59, 1971.
130. Mayfield DG: Alcohol problems in the aging patient. In Fann WE, Maddox GL (eds): Drug Issues in Geropsychiatry. Baltimore, Williams & Wilkins, 1974, pp 35–40.
131. Brody JA: Aging and alcohol abuse. J Am Geriat Soc 30:123-126, 1982.
132. Glatt MM, Rosin AJ, Jauhar P: Alcohol problems in the elderly. Age and Ageing 7 (suppl):64-66; (discussion) 67–71, 1978.
133. Sellers EM, Holloway MR: Drug kinetics and alcohol ingestion. Clin Pharmacokinet 3:440–452, 1978.
134. Hartford JT, Samorajski T: Alcoholism in the geriatric population. J Am Geriat Soc 30:18–24, 1982.
135. Rifkin H: Recognition and complications of diabetes in the older patient. J Am Geriat Soc 30 (suppl):S30–S35, 1982.
136. Ehrlich GE: Diagnosis and management of rheumatic disease in older patients. J Am Geriat Soc 30 (suppl): S45–S51, 1982.
137. Caruso I, Bianchi-Porro G: Gastroscopic evaluation of anti-inflammatory agents. Br Med J 280:75–78, 1980.
138. Torres VE: Present and future of the nonsteroidal anti-inflammatory drugs in nephrology. Mayo Clin Proc 57:389–393, 1982.
139. Ciabattoni G, Pugliese F, Cinotti GA, Patrono C: Renal effects of anti-inflammatory drugs. Eur J Rheumatol Inflamm 3:210–221, 1980.
140. Bunning RD, Barth WF: Sulindac: A potentially renal-sparing non-steroidal anti-inflammatory drug. JAMA 248:2864–2867, 1982.
141. Calin A: Non-steroidal anti-inflammatory drugs and frusemide-induced diuresis. Br Med J 283:1399–1400, 1981.

2 | Food Choices of the Elderly

Eleanor D. Schlenker

Medical advances in the control of infectious diseases and the decline in the infant death rate have brought about a dramatic increase in life expectancy in the United States.[1] Although the number of older individuals has increased proportionately, knowledge relating to the food choices and nutrient requirements of this age group is limited. Furthermore, evaluation of the food habits of the aged is extremely complex, as many factors beyond the control of older individuals may significantly affect their accessibility to food. These elements may include lack of money to purchase food, physical disability, isolation, or limited knowledge concerning adequate nutritional intake.[2] The impact of inadequate food intake on an individual whose nutritional status is already marginal as a result of physiologic factors relating to use of drugs or disease processes may be devastating to general health and lead to further disability. This chapter will focus on current knowledge regarding the food habits and food procurement problems of the aged as influenced by physiologic and socioeconomic factors, and on existing programs designed to alleviate these difficulties.

PHYSIOLOGIC FACTORS

Physiologic changes relating to both the normal aging process and degenerative disease may result in limitations in older individuals' ability to deal with their food needs. The most obvious implications of physical infirmity are the inability to leave one's home and shop for food and/or the inability to prepare adequate meals once food is brought into the home. Physical factors that may be less well recognized but that still exert a considerable effect on the food habits of the aged include loss of appetite and reduced sense of taste, which make eating less pleasurable. A therapeutic diet prescribed in the treatment of chronic disease may influence food intake both directly and indirectly since the older patient may lose interest in eating if favorite foods are deleted from the diet. Therefore, the health professional should become familiar not only with the medical records of older clients but also with their living situations and attitudes toward food.

Physical Disability

Chronic disease frequently results in functional disability of some degree. The most prevalent chronic conditions affecting the physical health of older persons include arthritis, hearing impairments, vision impairments, hypertension, and heart conditions.[3] These chronic problems may significantly impair an individual's ability to carry out food-related activities. Unfortunately, there has been no systematic attempt to define the impact of major or minor activity limitation on the food intake of the aged.

Food and Nutrient Intake   Available evidence points to the fact that chronic conditions as described above may seriously influence an individual's food pattern.[4,5] Exton-Smith,[4] reporting on 879 English aged living in their own homes, noted that in the group with the lowest intake of calories, about 20% had a serious chronic condition, such as failing vision or osteoarthritis, which impeded consumption and/or preparation of food. Similarly, Lonergan et al.[5] described two elderly patients with energy intakes less than one half the recommended level. One woman had diabetic retinopathy with severe osteoarthritis of the hip, and the other had poor vision and fixed flexion in both knees. Inasmuch as 38% of older persons in the United States suffer from arthritis of varying severity,[3] this relationship to nutrient intake should be explored further.

Several workers[5] investigated further the influence of particular disease states on nutrient intake among 212 men and 263 women, ages 62 to 90 years. Such conditions as visual acuity, congestive heart failure, reduced hip or knee movement, and stroke were not found to be associated with intakes of energy, protein, calcium, iron, ascorbic acid, or vitamin D. Men with chronic dyspnea or hearing loss, however, were more likely to have inadequate intakes of one or more nutrients. Women with mental illness, particularly dementia (defined on the basis of psychiatric examination), had significantly low intakes of five nutrients, indicative of malnutrition. (Specific nutrients were not defined.) The influence of age among these subjects, however, was not addressed.

Indirect evidence regarding chronic disease or disability and food intake comes from evaluations of older patients within geriatric facilities.[6,7] Evaluation of body build of 66 elderly patients in a long-stay hospital revealed no relationship between their current energy intake and skinfold thickness.[6] Contrary to what might have been anticipated, the body build of long-term patients appeared to be determined by their energy intake prior to admission. Among those patients, reduced skinfold thickness was most commonly found in those suffering disability from rheumatoid arthritis. Hurdle and Williams,[7] examining folic acid status in the aged, grouped patients according to general mobility and ability to "forage" and prepare food. Low serum folate was significantly related to the severity of the disability. In groups with mild as compared with severe impairment of mobility, 22% and 39%, respectively, had serum folate levels indicative of deficiency. That study also demonstrated the impact of psychologic outlook on food consumption. Two thirds of those diagnosed as having "no motivation" were folate deficient. Those investigators considered folate status to reflect food folate intake, rather than malabsorption of ingested folate.

In summary, persons with diminished mobility appear to consume less food and food of poorer nutritional quality than those better able to move about. This reduction in nutrient intake may lead to a further deterioration in physical status.

Food Procurement and Preparation   Limitation in physical activity that relates to general mobility can lead to problems in shopping and food procurement. In a study of elderly urban households,[8] 22% revealed health-related problems, such as poor eyesight, that might present difficulty in food shopping. As suggested by one writer,[9] the new, attractive supermarkets that offer a great variety of foods and are convenient for the young, able-bodied, and affluent may present one more disabling hurdle to the already-underprivileged aged. At the neighborhood grocery store, a telephone call could result in delivery of a food order.

If an automobile is not available for transportation, riding the bus or walking becomes a necessary alternative. Handling bundles of groceries on slippery sidewalks may prove impossible. Moreover, aged living in cold climates might, during the winter months, be shut in for a substantial number of days or even weeks. The inability to purchase fresh and nutritious food for such a period of time could significantly influence nutrient intake. Among rural elderly in southwestern Pennsylvania,[10] infrequent trips to the grocery store contributed to the low consumption of milk and subsequent deficient intakes of calcium and vitamin A. Lack of storage space[11] may also necessitate frequent shopping, with serious implications when shopping is impossible. For aged who must carry grocery bundles, light-weight dehydrated foods and packaged mixes may be selected in preference to heavier fresh, frozen, or canned items. Such substitutions may have a significant impact on the nutrient quality of the diet.

Older persons not having access to transportation are forced to shop at a store within walking distance. In rural areas, if there is a store within walking distance, it is a general store with a limited selection of items and sizes. Furthermore, in such stores, prices tend to be higher.[10] There may also be a similar problem in urban areas. As reported in one urban location, three neighborhood supermarkets closed in one year as a result of the development of a shopping mall at some distance.[9] A fourth, independently owned grocery store and meat market was replaced by a self-service convenience-type grocery. In that study, 20% of the older shoppers who walked to the store lived at a distance of eight or more blocks. Such individuals are dependent on neighbors, friends, or family members for transportation to a food store.

Various communities have developed different approaches for providing transportation for their older citizens. In some cases, van or bus service has been established to transport older persons to and from the store, and supermarkets cooperate in providing assistance with shopping for those requiring it. This assistance may include packaging small units for individuals living alone. Another possible alternative might be the delivery of grocery orders to housebound aged.

Another approach taken by aged with decreasing mobility in an effort to solve their food problem is the use of convenience or preprepared food items that require less effort in meal preparation. This trend was evident among 102 independent-living Kansas elderly who indicated significant modifications in their food habits over the preceding two years.[12] Frozen pot pies, frozen dinners, canned soups, and boxed desserts were consumed more frequently. Unless the convenience foods used provide the same levels of nutrients as the foods they are replacing, such practices may severely affect the nutrient quality of the diet. Highly processed foods are frequently low in content of trace minerals and such vitamins as folate, pyridoxine, and vitamin B_{12}. Moreover, such convenience items as frozen pies and dinners and canned soups tend to be high in sodium and fat content, which may also be detrimental to the diet of the older person.

State of Health

Chronic health problems may result in changes in the type and quantity of food consumed even in the absence of physical disability. Among Kansas aged,[12] the greater the number of reported changes in traditional food habits, the lower the nutritional scores. Food changes are frequently related to poor health, inactivity, and problems in preparing or procuring food. Some of these changes may have involved prescribed diets or limitations of dietary fat or sodium, as subjects consumed beef, liver, fresh and cured pork, and eggs less frequently. On the other hand, fruits and juices were consumed more frequently. According to another investigator,[13] older subjects commonly avoided high-fat and fried foods because they had been so advised by a physician.

Prescribed Diets   Estimates of the number of older individuals following physician-prescribed diets are varied. Among 303 noninstitutionalized Illinois aged 65 years of age and over, studied by Brown,[14] 43% were following prescribed diets. In general, the dietary modification involved restriction of fiber, carbohydrate, or fat. Dietary adequacy was not evaluated in respect to diet modification; however, nutrient intake among subjects was rather high. Seventy-three percent consumed more than 100% of the Recommended Dietary Allowance (RDA) for protein, riboflavin, and vitamins A and C. The two nutrients consumed at the lowest levels were calcium and niacin; 15% reported intakes less than two thirds of the RDA. Low levels of iron and thiamin were consumed by 7% and 11%, respectively, of persons interviewed. This report would suggest that prescribed diets need not result in dietary inadequacy. It should be pointed out, however, that these subjects were retired university employees, with an income and educational level above average.

Additional evidence relating prescribed diets and nutritional adequacy comes from the work of LeBovit and Baker.[15] Three in ten aged households surveyed in Rochester, New York, had at least one member following a modified diet in the treatment of organic disease, including diabetes, cardiovascular disease, gallbladder trouble, or gastrointestinal disorders. Contrary to what might have been anticipated, however, diseases requiring special diets did not appear to adversely affect the quality of the diet. In fact, no diabetic had a "poor" diet (containing less than two thirds the RDA for one or more nutrients). Inadequate diets were more likely to be associated with efforts at weight control. Among older women examined in Michigan, however, the reverse was true.[16] Those restricted in fiber-containing fruits and vegetables in the treatment of diverticular disease had low intakes of vitamins A and C. Since that time, however, dietary treatment for this condition has been altered.

Health-related changes in food choices were reported by 59 Michigan women (age range 58–89 years) studied by Johnson et al.[17] Forty-three percent of those subjects were following a modified diet recommended by their physician, including salt restriction, reduced fat or cholesterol, weight reduction, and diabetic regimens. An increase in consumption of fiber-containing foods was reported by 17%, whereas a similar number reduced fiber intake. These changes in fiber intake were based on medical advice. Specific nutrient intakes of these subjects were not reported.

In general, restricted foods tend to be those high in either fiber or fat content. Inasmuch as high-fiber foods, such as fruits, vegetables, and whole grains, are also good sources of many vitamins and trace minerals, the nutritional implications are of concern. Reducing the fat content of the diet may significantly affect the energy level of the diet, as fat is a concentrated source of calories.

Of greater concern for the older individual may be the psychologic effect of a modified diet. This effect may relate to a generalized misunderstanding of the time sequence of the regimen. Leslie[18] reported on a patient being treated for arthritis who had been advised to eat no meat, milk, cheese, or white bread, and to reduce the amount of butter and eggs consumed. After ten years, the patient continued to follow this diet and understandably suffered from anemia and osteomalacia.

Deletion from the diet of favorite or preferred foods, particularly those of religious or cultural significance, may further discourage the older individual with a limited appetite.[19] A recent marketing study[20] revealed that 56% of older adults were attempting to limit their use of salt and were considering purchase of a salt substitute. According to Brown,[14] 50% of elderly respondents selected foods on the basis of taste and personal enjoyment. A change in the accustomed flavor of foods may reduce interest in eating. North Carolina aged[21] who reported frequent problems with their diets had experienced significant changes in their food habits after age 50. An important component of any diet prescription for an aged patient should be personal counseling to allow for individual adaptation of the designated regimen.

Food Intolerance   The aging body is increasingly sensitive to digestive upset and food intolerance. Werner and Hambraeus[22] documented the increase in gastric symptoms as a function of age. Whereas less than 5% of subjects ages

20–25 years indicated abdominal distress or food intolerance, over 25% of persons over age 67 reported these problems. About 10% were fat intolerant. As suggested by these authors, fat intolerance may relate to decreased secretion of lipoprotein lipase, resulting in fecal (neutral) fat.

Furthermore, avoidance of gas-forming vegetables and fat was reported among older households in Rochester, New York,[15] and independent-living aged in Boston[13] and Michigan.[16] For the Rochester households,[15] the impact of food avoidance on the nutritional quality of the diet was slight, as few foods were involved. In fact, more households reporting avoidance of foods associated with discomfort had good diets (meeting 100% of the RDA for all nutrients). The total impact of avoidance of gas-forming, spicy, or fat-containing food on dietary quality is largely undefined. Johnson et al.[17] explored the issue of food avoidance in respect to dietary fiber intake. In that group of older women, 17% avoided cooked dried beans; 9%, onions; and 5%, cabbage. Analysis of those diets revealed that 21% of the total fiber was supplied by cooked vegetables and 19% by bread. This finding would suggest that avoidance of gas-forming vegetables would not significantly decrease fiber intake. Conversely, avoidance of fresh fruits and raw vegetables because of difficulties with mastication may impact on the fiber content of the diet.

Significant numbers of aged have also reported avoiding foods high in fat content. Elderly women (institutionalized) interviewed by Harrill et al.[19] described changes in their consumption of fatty or fried foods as well as "heavy" foods, such as pancakes or waffles. Twenty-two percent indicated that such foods caused digestive discomfort. Among 551 English elderly[23] who kept dietary records for seven days, 14% of the men and 25% of the women did not consume any fried foods during that period, and over half did not eat the fat on meat. Moreover, 15% of the men and 38% of the women did not add salt at the table.

This limitation of dietary fat raises questions relative to fatty acid and fat-soluble vitamin nutriture. Dietary fats are sources of linoleic acid, the essential fatty acid. A limited intake of fat coupled with possible problems in fat digestion and absorption could result in marginal nutritional status for the essential fatty acid. Similarly, a borderline vitamin A intake exacerbated by use of laxatives and only limited fat to aid in absorption could precipitate a vitamin A deficiency.

Efforts at Weight Control   A health-related problem that can have a disastrous effect on dietary quality is caloric balance to avoid or reduce weight gain. With the age-related decrease in basal metabolism and limitation in physical activity, the need to regulate caloric intake becomes essential.[2] Unfortunately, it may be difficult to evaluate food choices in order to maintain nutrient density as the number of calories consumed decreases. McClean et al.[24] addressed this problem, as four aged men in that study, with daily intakes below 1600 calories, were restricting energy in an effort to lose weight. Those authors noted that, contrary to the generally held opinion that older persons consume only tea, bread, butter, and biscuits, the overall quality of the diets of these men was generally satisfactory, with the exception of reduced calories and vitamin C. Among English aged examined by Lonergan,[23] 18% and 9% of the females and males, respectively, were following a weight-reduction regimen. Significant numbers of subjects were omitting sugar, potatoes, and alcohol from their diets, although many women reporting efforts at weight reduction still consumed sweets, cakes, and biscuits.

Indirect evidence of attempts to limit calorie intake comes from a study of food and television-viewing habits of independent-living aged. More than half of those subjects commented that they never consumed potato chips, soda, cupcakes, pretzels, beer, or popcorn.[25] Unfortunately, efforts at weight reduction were deleterious to the nutrient quality of the diet in older households in Rochester, New York.[15] Nearly one fifth of those consuming poor diets were attempting to lose weight. Specific deficiencies were not reported. Johnson et al.[17] noted that aged women limiting caloric intake had lowered intakes of dietary fiber.

A central issue to be considered in nutrition education of the aged is how to make wise choices on items to be deleted from the diet when caloric reduction becomes imperative. Exton-Smith and Stanton[26] evaluated the nutrient quality of diets, as caloric intake decreased from 2,074 to 1,674 calories in women of 71.8 and 89.9 years of age, respectively. In that study, nutrient intake declined as a result of changes in the quantity rather than the kinds of food consumed, nutrient density per 1,000 calories remained the same. However, foods high in protein and fat were consumed in lower amounts. Unfortunately, foods generous in protein and fat are also likely to contribute vitamins and minerals to the diet as well. As protein intake decreased from 63.0 to 47.8 g daily, calcium, iron, and vitamin C levels dropped from 924, 11.3, and 42 mg to 760, 8.0, and 29 mg, respectively. According to these authors, foods mainly carbohydrate in nature should be deleted first if caloric reduction is required. Levels of meat, fish, eggs, milk, and cheese should be maintained.

Nutrient Intake and Health Maintenance   Various investigators[4,26,27] have observed that aged persons in poor health consume less nutritionally adequate diets than those in better health. Among older Michigan women,[27] those considered to have good health and vitality tended to drink more milk and eat more vegetables, whole grains, cereals, and eggs than women classified as in poor health. An English survey[4] of 425 aged men and 454 aged women revealed that those whose general condition was judged to be "worse" than average on the basis of clinical examination consumed fewer calories than those of similar age judged to be "much better" or "better" than average. The low energy consumption of those in poor health could relate to reduced requirements imposed by limitation of physical activity.

Further evidence for a relationship between nutrient intake and state of health comes from Exton-Smith and Stanton.[26] In that instance, aged with better than average health consumed 12% of their calories as protein, whereas those with poorer-than-average health and of similar age consumed less than that amount. As noted previously, protein-rich-foods also tend to be rich in vitamins and minerals; therefore the overall quality of the diet may have been significantly improved in the above-average group. As concluded by those authors, although subjects in better health consume better-than-average diets, it cannot be assumed that diet influences health. The reverse might also be true in that persons in declining health are less able to maintain dietary adequacy.

Sensory Enjoyment of Food

Appetite   A physiologic factor that indirectly may lead to reduced food intake is loss of appetite and subsequent disinterest in eating. In a group of 526 English aged studied by Lonergan,[23] nearly half demonstrated no particular interest in the choice of foods in their diet, complaining that "all food tasted the same." Similarly, over half of 130 Bostonians[13] living in their own homes thought of eating as a necessary activity rather than as a pleasure. Appetites were reported as "good" by 67% and "fair" by 25% of aged persons living alone in Westchester, New York.[28]

Poor appetite may seriously affect the nutrient quality of the diet, as was suggested by a study of older households in Rochester, New York.[15] Sixteen percent of those with "poor" diets reported a lack of appetite, compared with 3% and 8% of those with "fair" or "good" diets, respectively. "Good" diets met or exceeded the RDA for all nutrients; "fair" diets fell between 67% and 100% of the RDA for all nutrients; and "poor" diets contained less than 67% of the RDA for one or more nutrients.

Health problems may also impair the appetite. Johnson et al.[17] reported that women with more health problems tended to have reduced caloric intakes and poor appetite. Inasmuch as many drugs prescribed in the treatment of chronic disease are known to reduce appetite,[29] decreased food intake may be a consequence in some aged patients.

Oral/Dental Problems   Reduced appetite may relate to age-associated changes in the oral cavity that make eating more difficult and less pleasurable. These changes may include reduced taste sensitivity, problems in swallowing, or inability to chew.[30] A factor closely associated with dentition and condition of the oral cavity is the sense of taste. Sensitivity to all four modalities—sweet, sour, salty, and bitter—begins to decline after age 55.[31,32] The perceived taste of food is also affected by the olfactory response. Healthy elderly subjects were less able to differentiate between simulated food odors than were younger individuals.[33] The generous use of salt by the older individual, generally discouraged by health practitioners, may represent an effort to strengthen this flavor when sensitivity has declined. This concept finds support in the work of Nizel,[30] who suggests that taste acuity for salt regresses as a result of gradual nerve degeneration of the epithelium.

Loss of teeth is another problem, as one half of all persons over the age of 65 are edentulous,[34] and only three fourths of these have either complete or partial dentures. Problems with mastication do not always, however, hinder consumption of a nutritious diet, as was suggested by an evaluation of 100 older persons in Westchester, New York.[28] In that study, 65 rated their ability to chew as "good," 11 as "fair," and 24 as "poor." Although 76 of the subjects wore dentures, only 4 related mastication to a change in food habits. Similarly, a survey of older households in Rochester, New York,[15] revealed that of subjects with poor, fair, and good diets, 5%, 6%, and 3%, respectively, reported difficulty with chewing. Healthy aged in rural Pennsylvania[35] demonstrated no influence of dentition on nutrient intake.

Individuals who do chew less efficiently may still maintain nutritional quality in their diets by selecting food requiring less mastication, as has been suggested by

Neill and Phillips,[36] who evaluated the masticatory performance and food intake of 53 elderly men, with a mean age of 78 years. Efficiency in mastication was measured by the volume of chewed food passing through a mesh screen of given pore size after a certain number of chews. Those subjects with the most efficient mastication had the highest food intake relative to total calories, carbohydrate, fat, and animal and vegetable protein, as compared with those with lower masticatory performance scores. Although these differences were not significant, this trend bears further investigation. In this study, individuals with relatively poor masticatory performance still had protein and calorie intakes well within recommended levels. It must be recognized, however, that these subjects, residents in a retirement home with high dietary standards, had access to various meat and protein dishes well cooked and attractively served. Such a variety may not be available to individuals living in their homes.

Other investigators have reported relationships between oral status and nutrient consumption.[13,23,26] Protein intake (gm/kg body weight) was inversely correlated with chewing efficiency among 130 healthy aged studied by Davidson et al.[13] Evidence that ability to chew may be involved in ascorbic acid nutriture comes from Exton-Smith and Stanton.[26] They described two elderly subjects in London who, having only a few teeth and no dentures, avoided "hard or tough foods," such as fruits and vegetables. As might be anticipated, both women had low intakes of ascorbic acid. Ill-fitting dentures or lack of dentures was given as one reason for limited consumption of fresh fruit by older men interviewed by Lonergan.[23] These studies relating dentition and intake of ascorbic acid-rich foods may not reflect the present availability of juices with high ascorbic acid content. Nevertheless, this area may require surveillance on the part of health professionals working with edentulous aged.

The most critical nutritional aspect of poor dentition among the aged may be their inability to select from a variety of foods and to chew favorite foods.[37,38] Full dentures properly fitted, however, may allow the consumption of many food types. The eating patterns of 279 veterans were studied before and after the men were fitted with dentures.[39] When dentures were worn for eating, subjects consumed less bread and more crisp raw vegetables. There were no measurable differences in the consumption of milk, protein foods, ascorbic acid-rich foods, green and yellow vegetables, and other vegetables and fruits. Eating patterns were more related to food availability than dentures, as those subjects provided with nutritionally adequate foods within a domiciliary had improved diets, as compared with those living at home.

In planning diets for the older person with limited ability to chew, it should be noted that even fresh fruits and vegetables and meats can be consumed if cut into small pieces. Eggs and selected dairy products are excellent sources of high-quality protein.

Home-Delivered Meals Program

As suggested above, disease and related disability may contribute significantly to a person's inability to handle meal preparation. It has been reported that at least 10% of persons over the age of 65 have difficulty preparing a hot meal for themselves.[40] In order to provide for aged who have disabilities, various community and nonprofit agencies have attempted to develop programs that provide meals delivered to the home.

The first Meals on Wheels program in the United States was begun in Philadelphia in 1954;[41] by 1971, over 170 meal delivery programs had been established.[42] In Great Britain, home-delivered meals are provided by government service agencies. Unfortunately, all such programs are less likely to be organized in rural areas, where persons live at some distance from one another and resources are less accessible.

In general, meal delivery programs provide one hot meal each day, five days per week. The hot meal is delivered at noon and may be accompanied by a cold supper to be consumed later. Special diets (i.e., diabetic, low sodium) may be available, depending on the agency supplying the meals. Meal delivery services operated by hospitals or nursing homes usually include this option. Guidelines developed by the National Council on the Aging[43] suggest that each delivered meal provide at least one third of the daily recommended level of nutrients; however, adherence to this guide by community programs not receiving federal funds is strictly voluntary. In any case, the delivered meals do not provide all nutrients needed for the day; moreover, meals are not delivered on weekends or holidays. Therefore, recipients are required to have another source of either meals or groceries.

At present, objective data describing either the aged population served by home-delivered meals or the nutritional impact of these meals on their dietary pattern are limited. Available data, however, would support the concept that the older the individual, the greater the vulnerability to difficulty with food preparation. Piper et al.,[44] conducting a survey of 16 meal delivery programs, reported the median age of recipients as 78. Ninety percent of those receiving meals were above age 60, and 40% were at least age 80. Furthermore, meal recipients were more likely to be women than men.[44] This finding could relate to the fact that in older age groups, women outnumber men.

Living arrangements and accessibility to cooking facilities also influence the dependence of an aged person on home-delivered meals. According to one report,[45] a majority of recipients lived alone in a single room. Other writers[44] indicated that 70% of recipients lived alone, although eight out of ten had kitchen facilities. Meals on Wheels may also be utilized as a temporary, short-term food service when necessitated by temporary health conditions.[46]

The actual nutrient content of home-delivered meals in the United States is not well defined. Henry,[47] describing a New York program, indicated that the delivery, consisting of hot meal and cold supper, provided three fourths of the nutrient needs of a 65-year-old male. Several English investigators,[26,48–50] however, have evaluated the impact of home-delivered meals on total dietary intake. According to one report,[48] about two thirds of the vitamin A and three fourths of the ascorbic acid consumed on delivery days were supplied by the home-delivered meal. Furthermore, caloric intake increased (about 120 calories) on days when a meal was delivered, as compared with days when all food was obtained from other sources.[49] Another nutrient that has been evaluated in home-delivered meals is potassium.[50] In that study, 32% of the subjects had daily potassium intakes below 2,000 mg

(50mEq), and the home-delivered meal contained an average of only 1,100 mg (28 mEq).

One factor that strongly influences the total impact of a meal delivery program is the number of days on which meals are provided. An evaluation of the food habits of 107 London aged[51] revealed that a meal delivery schedule of less than four days per week resulted in no significant contribution to the overall diet. It should also be pointed out that over 80% of those individuals had adequate meals provided by neighbors when no meal was delivered. The remainder did have markedly reduced nutrient intakes on days when no meal was available from either source. In rural areas, where neighbors may be at some distance, nutrient intake may be significantly lower on nondelivery days.

Although the nutrient quality of the home-delivered meals may be excellent, this quality is of no value unless the food is actually consumed. A food preference questionnaire administered to participants in an Ohio program indicated that meat, desserts, milk, and potatoes were among foods enjoyed the most; fish was enjoyed the least.[45] In a London program, wastage was reported as "high."[51] Reasons given for nonconsumption included too large portions, items difficult to chew, unpalatability, and poor cooking.

Another factor that may influence the acceptability of home-delivered meals is the established meal pattern of the recipient. This factor was suggested by a survey of 200 meal recipients in Australia[52]; only 43% ate the entire meal as soon as it was delivered at noon, and 15% discarded a portion of the meal. The others consumed either the whole or a portion of the meal at a later time. This would point to the importance of available refrigeration for the person receiving home-delivered meals.

Rapidly increasing fuel costs raise serious questions relating to the expansion and/or continuation of daily meal delivery. Innovative approaches for providing meals to homebound aged might include a weekly delivery of several frozen meals to be heated as needed, or the delivery of groceries for meal preparation. A recent demonstration project involved the mail delivery of freeze-dried foods (requiring simple heating procedures) to homebound aged.[53] Respondents found the meals to be convenient, easy to prepare, and tasty, and a majority expressed a desire to continue in the program. Nutrient evaluation of the foods was not reported. New approaches for nutritional support in home care need to be explored.

SOCIOECONOMIC FACTORS

Many social, psychologic, and economic factors may influence the food patterns of the older individual. Changes in life-style and family situation can result in emotional upheaval and subsequent frustration. Retirement from full-time employment can lead to diminished feelings of self-worth, disruption of the daily schedule, and irregular food patterns. The bereaved widow who may be living and eating alone for the first time in her life may not put forth the effort to cook adequate meals. The elderly man who has never had to prepare his own food may not have the resources to cope with this responsibility. Finally, spiraling inflation creates continuing financial anxiety for older persons on fixed incomes. All of these factors can contribute to problems in food selection.[2]

Nutrition Knowledge

Poor food choices by older persons may relate to a lack of information regarding nutritional needs and nutrient sources. A consumer survey[54] revealed that age and education were significantly related to nutrition knowledge. Those with low nutrition knowledge tended to be older (over age 50) and came from the lower socioeconomic group. This finding may be related to the limited sources of information utilized by older consumers. For example, 70% of older shoppers (110 households) from a metropolitan area indicated their primary sources of information regarding food products to be newspapers or television.[8] Other aged consumers, asked to name sources of nutrition information that had been most helpful to them in the past, listed television, physicians, magazine articles, and cookbooks. Food labels were infrequently used to obtain nutrition information.[55]

Meal Pattern/Leisure Time

Inasmuch as retirement places fewer demands on one's time, attention has focused on the meal patterns of older individuals. Reports suggest that a significant number consume less than three meals each day.[15,25,56,57] The meal most frequently omitted was at midday, although many did not have breakfast regularly. For some elderly, the two-meal pattern consisted of a late morning brunch and another meal in late afternoon. Limiting the number of meals each day may represent an effort at reducing calorie intake. Another study[28] confirms that many retired persons consume their main meal at noon. This pattern has important implications for both congregate and home-delivered meals programs that serve at noon.

Many older persons also eat between meals. Among 504 aged interviewed in New York,[15,25] nearly half reported snacking. In many instances this food was consumed in the evening. Of major concern is the type of food consumed as snacks, particularly if these snacks are to replace missed meals. Pao[56] found the most frequent snack item for both aged men and women was coffee. Other foods reported by men included milk, fruit, and sweet baked items, whereas women frequently chose sweet baked items. Some snacks among Rochester aged consisted of only beer or wine.[15] Clancy,[25] interviewing 47 retired persons, found a significant positive correlation between the percentage of calories contributed by snack foods and the number of hours of television watched daily. Moreover, television viewing in the evening was positively related to both total fat and calorie intake. Unfortunately, the higher the percentage of calories consumed as snacks, the poorer the general nutrient quality of the diet. This finding, relating snacking and television viewing with reduced nutrient quality, has serious implications regarding the nutriture of the aged. For many older individuals, particularly those with limited mobility, television is a favored pastime. Inasmuch as this activity does present an ideal environment for snacking, an emphasis should be placed on the selection of nutritious snacks.

One report[15] does suggest that snacking can have a positive effect on the diet. Milk or other dairy products and fruit were popular choices between meals in those older subjects. In that study, the calcium content of snacks was higher than that of any meal, and the ascorbic acid intake from snacks was almost as high as that consumed at breakfast. Older persons might be encouraged to consider snacks as part of the total daily pattern and include highly nutritious items, particularly in light of the need to control calorie intake.

Social Isolation

Food frequently fulfills social and psychologic needs relating to companionship, comfort, and sense of personal and family well-being. Various investigators[13,15,25,55,58,59] have related the degree of social interaction and level of nutrients consumed. Dietary adequacy was significantly related to the social participation scores of 47 New York aged.[25] In that study, social participation included visiting out of the house on a daily basis or having friends visit at least weekly. Those individuals with higher levels of social participation reported significantly greater intakes of calories, iron, thiamin, and riboflavin, as well as higher dietary scores. Dietary scores were calculated on the basis of the number of nutrients present in the diet at two thirds or more of the recommended level.

Further evidence that eating with others increases food consumption comes from the work of Grotkowski and Sims[55] with urban aged. Not only did subjects who ate regularly with others consume more calories, but the quality of the diet improved as well, with increased intakes of iron, niacin, ascorbic acid, thiamin, and protein. In those subjects, socioeconomic status also related to nutrients consumed with others. Individuals in a higher socioeconomic bracket were more likely to entertain at mealtime or to eat in restaurants. Similar findings relating degree of social contact and nutrient intake were reported for elderly in Dublin.[58] Those individuals living with relatives had improved overall dietary intakes as compared with those who lived alone but obtained some meals at a day center. The subjects who resided alone and never shared meals consumed less protein, iron, and ascorbic acid, with fewer calories. A survey of 1,771 English aged[59] over 60 years of age revealed that men and women living alone ate less of those foods requiring some preparation. Social isolation may also influence the variety of foods consumed. The "variety score," assessed by totaling the number of different foods consumed, was significantly lower for Boston aged living alone.[13]

Differences in nutrient intake between one- and two-person households may relate to a single-female versus single-male household. Among 283 older households in Rochester, New York,[15] 45%, 48%, and 43% of the husband-wife, single-male and single-female households, respectively, had good diets (meeting or exceeding the RDA for all nutrients). Conversely, 39% of the single-male households and 29% of the single-female households had poor diets (less than two thirds the RDA for one or more nutrients). Only 25% of the husband-wife households had poor diets. Single men tended to consume generous amounts of dairy products, and 83% met the RDA for calcium. Single women tended to have low intakes of iron-rich foods. Single persons age 75 or over were particularly vulnerable to poor nutrient intake. Various investigators[4,10,59] have commented on the nutritional problems of older men living alone, particularly in relation to vitamins A, C, and folic acid. Among the 100 aged living alone interviewed by Jordan et al.,[28] the food group most frequently omitted from the diet was green and yellow vegetables. Reported findings may relate to the relative degree of isolation. Although individuals live alone, they may still interact with neighbors or friends at mealtime or possibly eat outside their home.

Economic Status

Although some older persons may have sufficient funds to live comfortably and free of worry, the great majority are caught by spiraling inflation and fixed income. The level of income frequently influences the food choices available to the aged person. Among 100 aged in Westchester, New York,[28] 20% reported changes in food habits for economic reasons. Similarly, decreased consumption of meat reported by Boston aged was related to diminished income.[13] Available evidence would suggest that low-income aged have diets poorer in nutrient quality than median- or high-income aged.[35,55,60] Grotkowski and Sims[55] reported lower intakes of calories, protein, and fat for urban aged with lower incomes. Aged residing in downtown urban hotels (single-room occupancy) were observed to subsist on coffee and doughnuts, the only foods they could afford.[60]

The study of dietary adequacy and economic parameters may be approached on the basis of the amount of money spent for food each week.[15,35,61] Among 264 English aged living at home, the weekly food expenditure proved to be a significant variable in identifying elderly most vulnerable to poor nutrient intake.[61] This relationship was also examined by Guthrie et al.[35] in rural Pennsylvanians. One-person households identified as low income on the basis of eligibility for food stamps had food expenditures on both a per-week and per-month basis only half that of non-low-income households. Relative to nutrient quality, the low-income subjects had significantly lower intakes of protein, iron, and riboflavin and consumed less meat and fruit. Diets were evaluated further, taking into consideration not only eligibility for food stamps but actual enrollment in the food stamp program. Among food stamp recipients, 36% consumed less than two thirds the RDA for calories; among low-income aged not receiving food stamps, this measure was 62%. Protein intake was below two thirds the recommended level for 28% of the food stamp recipients as compared with 47% of eligible nonrecipients. In the case of iron intake, these values were 7% and 32%, respectively. The number of food stamp recipients falling seriously below the recommended levels of these three nutrients did not differ significantly from that observed in the non-low-income group. This finding would point to the importance of food aid programs in maintaining nutritional health among the aged.

Money spent for food was also an indicator of dietary quality among older households in Rochester, New York.[15] In that study, households were classified according to food expenditures: (1) less than the U.S. Department of Agriculture low-cost food plan; (2) between the low-cost and liberal food plan; and (3) exceeding the liberal food plan. By this evaluation, 75% of those with poor diets spent less than the value of the low-cost plan for food. Conversely, over 50% of those with good diets were spending more than the liberal food plan estimate. It should be noted, however, that a few households spending liberal amounts of money on food had poor diets, and conversely, several (5%) managed to obtain good diets at low cost. According to these findings, education regarding food selection may improve a low-income diet to some extent; however, money available for food is still a significant factor.

Several national studies[62,63] have attempted to examine nutrient intake patterns in persons over age 60. Unfortunately, the number of subjects in this age cohort was limited. In the Ten-State Nutrition Survey 1968–1970, dietary intake was not strongly related to income.[62] In general, individuals from states classified as low income had lesser nutrient intakes than those in states considered to be higher in income, although persons age 60 and over appeared as a group to be at nutritional risk. Dietary levels of iron, protein, and thiamin related to total caloric intake, whereas vitamin C and riboflavin reflected the selection of particular foods rich in those nutrients.

According to the Health and Nutrition Examination Survey, aged having incomes above the poverty level had higher intakes of calories, protein, calcium, iron, vitamin A, and ascorbic acid than those with incomes below the poverty level.[63] Persons with lower incomes had mean intakes of iron (9.57 mg) and calcium (583 mg) below recommended levels. For higher-income individuals, these values were 11.41 and 666 mg, respectively. Unfortunately, these data are not separated according to sex.

Available evidence would suggest that level of income has serious implications for the nutritional adequacy of the diet consumed by older individuals. As their economic situation becomes precarious, the dietary consequences may be considerable.

Nutrition Program for Older Americans/Congregate Meals

The federally funded Nutrition Program for Older Americans (NPOA) was designed to provide low-cost, nutritionally adequate meals in a congregate setting for individuals age 60 and over. Authorized under the Older Americans Act of 1965, the NPOA is targeted to reach those who do not eat adequate meals because of limited income, disability, or lack of incentive to prepare adequate meals.[64] To fulfill this mandate, nutrition sites have been established that serve a hot meal, usually at noon, designed to provide at least one third of the daily recommended dietary needs of this age group. In urban areas, meals are usually served at least five days each week; in small communities and rural areas, meals may be served two to four days per week. An important component of the NPOA is socialization, and nutrition sites may be established in churches, community centers, public housing, or other public facilities. Transportation to the nutrition site may be provided for those in need. The impact of the NPOA is suggested by the fact that about 32 million meals were served at 12,500 nutrition sites in 1980. Over 3 million persons participated in the program.[65]

Although the NPOA may provide only a limited number of meals per week to each participant, available evidence does suggest that participation improves the overall dietary intake of the individual.[66-68] According to a report describing 547 NPOA participants in central Missouri, daily food records including an NPOA meal contained a significantly higher percentage of the RDA for energy, protein, calcium, riboflavin and niacin than those obtained on nonparticipation days.[66] This finding may relate to the inclusion of protein-rich foods, including a cup of milk, as part of the NPOA meal pattern.

The frequency of attendance is also a significant factor when estimating the impact of the NPOA on the food intake of participants. Evaluation of Missouri subjects who were (1) no longer participating at the time of the study, (2) participated irregularly (less than two times per week), or (3) participated regularly (two to five times per week) revealed that consumption of vitamin A and ascorbic acid-rich foods was significantly greater for those who attended even irregularly.[68] Among females, 41% and 55% of the nonparticipants and irregular participants, respectively, failed to consume an adequate number of servings of vitamin A-rich vegetables, as compared with only 26% of the regular participants. These findings would point to the importance of the vegetables and fruits served within the NPOA meal, as these foods are less likely to be consumed at home. This conclusion is further supported by the findings of Pelcovits,[57] who conducted 24-hour recall studies on 3,500 aged before their involvement in the NPOA. At that time, 34% had no fruit, 18% no vegetable, and 20% no milk or milk product on the day they were interviewed.

Even irregular participation in the NPOA appears to improve the quality of the diet of participants. Health professionals working with older persons at nutritional risk might direct them to the NPOA in their community.

GENERAL CONSIDERATIONS

As suggested in this paper, many factors may hinder the older individual from consuming a nutritionally adequate diet. Although nutrition surveys[69] of older persons frequently report mean nutrient intakes that are adequate when compared to current standards, many individuals are seriously lacking in particular nutrients. The nutrients most likely to be deficient in the older subject's diet are calories and calcium. In the Ten-State Survey,[62] over half of the respondents failed to meet the recommended level of calories. Among independent-living Missouri aged,[68] about 25% consumed less than two thirds the RDA for calories. An intake at least two thirds the RDA is generally considered to be adequate. Guthrie et al.[35] noted in 109 aged studied in rural Pennsylvania that 55% of the men and 42% of the women had less than 67% of the RDA for calories. This finding may reflect efforts at weight control and raises questions concerning the current recommended levels of energy intake.

Many studies,[4,13,15,35,62,63,69] have reported less-than-adequate levels of dietary calcium consumed in the aged. This problem is particularly serious in women, who appear to have only limited consumption of dairy products. Among rural Pennsylvanians,[35] nearly two thirds of all subjects interviewed had less-than-adequate (<67% of the RDA) intakes of this nutrient. In the Ten-State Survey,[62] over 33% of all subjects consumed less than 400 mg of calcium daily (RDA = 800 mg). Health professionals need to emphasize the nutritional value of milk and dairy products to individuals of all ages.

Generous use of selected dairy products may also contribute high-quality protein to the diet at relatively low cost. Although mean intakes of protein were more than adequate in many studies,[13,15,35,62,63,69] Guthrie et al.[35] reported protein intakes below two thirds that recommended in 29% of respondents. Over half of those interviewed in low-income states included in the Ten-State Survey[62] did not consume 1 g/kg body weight as recommended. Protein intake may be of particular concern among low-income aged.

Various investigators[13,15,35,62,63,68,69] have reported low iron intakes in older persons. Ten percent to 20% of rural Missouri[68] and Pennsylvania[35] aged consumed less than 6.7 mg (two thirds the RDA) of iron daily. This finding was also true for 40% of independent-living Bostonians studied by Davidson et al.[13] The majority of both men and women participating in a national survey[62] had less-than-recommended levels of iron. This finding might not have been anticipated in light of the highly fortified cereal products now available, which provide 10 mg of iron per serving. The biological availability of these iron forms, however, is not clearly understood.

Many older individuals have limited consumption of fruits and vegetables, particularly vitamin A- and vitamin C-rich varieties. Two thirds of the rural Pennsylvanians interviewed by Guthrie et al.[35] had less than 67% of the recommended level of vitamin A, and nearly half were below this level of vitamin C. In the Ten-State Survey,[62] Spanish-American aged were particularly low in vitamin A; one third of all subjects in that study were low in ascorbic acid. The impact of dental problems on dietary levels of vitamins A and C has been addressed.

Despite the widespread use of enriched breads and cereals, low intakes of the B complex vitamins (i.e., thiamin, riboflavin, and niacin) are common in the aged. Various investigators[62,63,69] have reported that 33% to 50% of older subjects have less-than-adequate dietary levels of these nutrients. Some older persons may limit use of carbohydrate foods as an effort at weight control. Consumption of whole-grain and enriched breads and cereals should be encouraged in this age group.

In summary, the nutrient intakes of many older persons are less than desirable. The factors relating to these food choices are both varied and complex. Inasmuch as each older person is faced with a unique set of physical and environmental circumstances, solutions must be explored on an individual basis. Whenever possible, the client should be encouraged to take advantage of appropriate community services designed to provide nutritional support.

REFERENCES

1. Metropolitan Life Insurance Company: Expectation of life in the United States at new high. Stat Bull Metropol Life Insur Co 61(4):13–15, 1980.
2. Stare FJ: Three score and ten plus more. J Am Geriatr Soc 25:529–533, 1977.
3. National Council on the Aging: Fact Book on Aging: A Profile of America's Older Population. Washington, National Council on the Aging, 1978.
4. Exton-Smith AN, Chairman, Panel on Nutrition of the Elderly: A Nutrition Survey of the Elderly. London, Her Majesty's Stationary Office, 1972.
5. Lonergan ME, Milne JS, Maule MM, Williamson J: A dietary survey of older people in Edinburgh. Br J Nutr 34:517–527, 1975.
6. MacLennan WJ, Martin P, Mason BJ: Energy intake, disability, disease and skinfold thickness in a long-stay hospital. Geront Clin 17:173–180, 1975.
7. Hurdle AD, Williams TC: Folic-acid deficiency in elderly patients admitted to hospital. Br Med J 2:202–205, 1966.
8. Mason JB, Bearden WO: Profiling the shopping behavior of elderly consumers. Gerontologist 18:454–461, 1978.
9. Sherman EM, Brittan MR: Contemporary food gatherers: A study of food shopping habits of an elderly urban population. Gerontologist 13:358–364, 1973.
10. Rawson IG, Weinburg EI, Herold JA, Holtz J: Nutrition of rural elderly in southwestern Pennsylvania. Gerontologist 18:24–29, 1978.
11. Rountree JL, Tinklin GL: Food beliefs and practices of selected senior citizens. Gerontologist 15:537–540, 1975.
12. Clarke M, Wakefield LM: Food choices of institutionalized vs. independent-living elderly. J Am Diet Assoc 66:600–604, 1975.
13. Davidson CS, Livermore J, Anderson P, Kaufman S: The nutrition of a group of apparently healthy aging persons. Am J Clin Nutr 10:181–199, 1962.
14. Brown EL: Factors influencing food choices and intake. Geriatrics 31:89–92, 1976.
15. LeBovit C, Baker DA: Food Consumption and Dietary Levels of Older Households in Rochester, New York. Home Economics Research Report No. 25. Washington, United States Department of Agriculture, 1965.
16. Schlenker ED: Nutritional status of older women. Ph.D. thesis. East Lansing, Michigan State University, 1976.
17. Johnson CK, Kolasa K, Chenoweth W, Bennink M: Health, laxation, and food habit influences on fiber intake of older women. J Am Diet Assoc 77:551–557, 1980.
18. Leslie J: Nutrition and diet: The elderly. Nurs Mirror 145(8):31–33, 1977.
19. Harrill I, Erbes C, Schwartz C: Observations on food acceptance by elderly women. Gerontologist 16:349–355, 1976.
20. Schiffman LG: Sources of information for the elderly. J Adv Res 11:33–37, 1971.
21. Learner RM, Kivett VR: Discriminators of perceived dietary adequacy among the rural elderly. J Am Diet Assoc 78:330–337, 1981.
22. Werner I, Hambraeus L: The digestive capacity of elderly people. In Carlson LA (ed): Nutrition in Old Age. Uppsala, Almqvist & Wiksell, 1972.
23. Lonergan ME: Nutritional survey of the elderly. Nutrition (London) 25:30–36, 1971.
24. McClean H, Weston R, Beaven DW, Riley CG: Nutrition of elderly men living alone. 1. Intakes of energy and nutrients. NZ Med J 84:305–309, 1976.
25. Clancy KL: Preliminary observations on media use and food habits of the elderly. Gerontologist 15:529–532, 1975.
26. Exton-Smith AN, Stanton BR: Report of an Investigation into the Dietary of Elderly Women Living Alone. Cambridge, England, Pendragon Press, 1965.

27. Ohlson MA, Roberts PH, Joseph SA, Nelson PM: Dietary practices of 100 women from 40 to 75 years of age. J Am Diet Assoc 24:286–291, 1948.

28. Jordan M, Kepes M, Hayes RB, Hammond W: Dietary habits of persons living alone. Geriatrics 9:230–232, 1954.

29. Baker CE: Physicians' Desk Reference, 34th ed. Oradell, NJ, Medical Economics Company, 1980.

30. Nizel AE: Role of nutrition in the oral health of the aging patient. Dent Clin North Am 20:569–584, 1976.

31. Glanville EV, Kaplan AR, Fischer R: Age, sex and taste sensitivity. J Gerontol 19:474–478, 1964.

32. Schiffman SS, Hornack K, Reilly D: Increased taste thresholds of amino acids with age. Am J Clin Nutr 32:1622–1627, 1979.

33. Schiffman SS, Pasternak M: Decreased discrimination of food odors in the elderly. J Gerontol 34:73–79, 1979.

34. United States Department of Health, Education and Welfare, Vital and Health Statistics: Edentulous Persons, United States. DHEW Publication No. (HRA) 74-1516, Series 10, No. 89. Rockville, Md., United States Public Health Service, 1974.

35. Guthrie HA, Black K, Madden JP: Nutritional practices of elderly citizens in rural Pennsylvania. Gerontologist 12:330–335, 1972.

36. Neill DJ, Phillips HIB: Masticatory performance, dental state, and dietary intake of a group of elderly army pensioners. Br Dent J 128:581–585, 1970.

37. Heath MR: Dietary selection by elderly persons related to dental state. Br. Dent J 132:145–148, 1972.

38. Chinn AB: Some problems of nutrition in the aged. JAMA 162:1511–1513, 1956.

39. Anderson EL: Eating patterns before and after dentures. J Am Diet Assoc 58:421–426, 1971.

40. Grant J: The feeding of the elderly in their own homes: Defining the need. Proc Nutr Soc 27:35–40, 1968.

41. Keller MD, Smith CE: Meals on Wheels, 1960. Geriatrics 16:237–247, 1961.

42. United States Department of Health, Education and Welfare: Home-Delivered Meals. A National Directory. SRS-AOA Publication No. 194. Washington, United States Government Printing Office, 1971.

43. National Council on the Aging: Home-delivered meals for the ill, handicapped and elderly. Am J Pub Hlth 55(suppl):1–86, 1965.

44. Piper GM, Frank B, Thorner RM: Survey of home-delivered meals. Pub Hlth Rep 80:432–436, 1965.

45. Williams IF, Smith CE: Home-delivered meals for the aged and handicapped. J Am Diet Assoc 35:146–149, 1959.

46. Ford CS, Kaplan J, Gremling G: Home-delivered meals help aged and ill live independently. Hospitals 42:80–83, 1968.

47. Henry CE: Feeding elderly people in their homes. J Am Diet Assoc 35:149–151, 1959.

48. Davies L, Hastrop K, Bender AE: Methodology of a survey on meals on wheels. Mod Geriatr 3:385–388, 1973.

49. Davies L, Hastrop K, Bender AE: The energy benefit of meals on wheels. Mod Geriatr 4:220–226, 1974.

50. Davies L, Hastrop K, Bender AE: Potassium intake of the elderly. Mod Geriatr 3:482–488, 1973.

51. Stanton BR: Feeding the elderly, meals on wheels in London. J NZ Diet Assoc 26:11–13, 1972.

52. Barker RA, Martin J: Feeding the elderly. 1. The Auckland meals on wheels service. J

NZ Diet Assoc 26:10–11, 1972.

53. Rhodes L: NASA food technology. A method for meeting the nutritional needs of the elderly. Gerontologist 17:333–340, 1977.
54. Fusillo AE, Beloian AM: Consumer nutrition knowledge and self-reported food shopping behavior. Am J Pub Hlth 67:846–850, 1977.
55. Grotkowski ML, Sims LS: Nutritional knowledge, attitudes, and dietary practices of the elderly. J Am Diet Assoc 72:499–505, 1978.
56. Pao E: Food patterns of the elderly. Family Economics Review, United States Department of Agriculture, December, 1971, pp 16–19.
57. Pelcovits J: Nutrition to meet the human needs of older Americans. J Am Diet Assoc 60:297–300, 1972.
58. Wilson CN, Nolan C: The diets of elderly people in Dublin. Ir J Med Sci 3:345–355, 1970.
59. Bransby ER, Osborne B: Social and food survey of elderly, living alone or as married couples. Br J Nutr 7:160–180, 1953.
60. Abrams M: The SRO elderly from the perspective of a hotel owner. In The Invisible Elderly. Washington, National Council on the Aging, 1976.
61. Caird FI, Judge TB, Macleod C: Pointers to possible malnutrition in the elderly at home. Geront Clin 17:47–54, 1975.
62. United States Department of Health, Education and Welfare, Health Services and Mental Health Administration: Ten-State Nutrition Survey 1968–1970. 5. Dietary. DHEW Publication No. (HSM) 72-8133. Atlanta, Center for Disease Control, 1972.
63. United States Department of Health, Education and Welfare, Public Health Service: Preliminary Findings of the First Health and Nutrition Examination Survey, United States, 1971–1972. Dietary Intake and Biochemical Findings. Rockville, National Center for Health Statistics, 1974.
64. United States Department of Health, Education and Welfare: Older Americans Act of 1965, As Amended. DHEW Publication No. (OHD) 76-20170. Washington, United States Government Printing Office, 1976.
65. United States Department of Health and Human Services: National Summary of States Performance Fiscal Year 1980. Washington, Administration on Aging, Office of Program Operations, 1981. (Courtesy J Carlin, Regional Nutritionist, Boston.)
66. Kohrs MB, O'Hanlon P, Eklund D: Title VII. Nutrition Program for the Elderly. 1. Contribution to one day's dietary intake. J Am Diet Assoc 72:489–492, 1978.
67. Kohrs MB: The Nutrition Program for Older Americans. J Am Diet Assoc 75:543–546.
68. Kohrs MB, Nordstrom J, Plowman EL, et al.: Association of participation in a nutritional program for the elderly with nutritional status. Am J Clin Nutr 33:2643–2656, 1980.
69. O'Hanlon P, Kohrs MB: Dietary studies of older Americans. Am J Clin Nutr 31:1257–1269, 1978.

3 | Food Effects on Drug Absorption in the Elderly

C.T. Viswanathan
Peter G. Welling

Most systemically acting drugs are taken by the oral route. The resulting drug levels in the circulation, and hence their therapeutic effect, are influenced by the efficiency with which the drug is absorbed from the gastrointestinal (GI) tract, and also by the rate at which absorption occurs.

The rate and extent to which orally administered drugs are absorbed from the GI tract are generally established in clinical trials using healthy, young, fasted individuals. The relevance of such data to elderly patients is uncertain. It becomes less certain if one considers that such patients frequently ingest their medication at mealtimes, the meal acting as a convenient reminder. A large number of studies have shown that the presence of food in the GI tract, or changes in accompanying fluid volumes, can have a marked and often unpredictable effect on drug absorption.[1-3]

Most reported studies have been carried out in younger patients or volunteers, and little information is available regarding drug-food or fluid volume-drug interactions in elderly patients or on the possible clinical significance of these interactions.

The purpose of this review is to consider the influence that food, specific dietary components, and also different fluid volumes may have on oral drug availability in the elderly in the light of known interactions that have been reported, predominantly in younger individuals, and changes in the physiology of the GI system of the older patient.

INFLUENCE OF AGE ON THE GASTROINTESTINAL TRACT

A number of changes occur in the physiology of the human GI tract in the older patient.[4,5,6,7] The pH of saliva shifts from slightly acidic to somewhat alkaline, esophageal peristalsis decreases, and muscles of the lower esophagus become weaker. Atrophic gastritis is more common than in younger patients,[5] secretion of hydrochloric acid is reduced in older patients, and achlorhydria may develop[8,9,10] possibly leading to reduced absorption of iron and vitamin B_{12}.[5]

The mucosal surface area of the small intestine decreases with age, mean villous height being reduced and the breadth increased.[11] Further changes in the intestinal mucosa may occur as a result of the use of laxatives in older patients.[12,13]

Gastric motility decreases with age, and this decrease may affect the absorption of substances that are unstable at acidic pH. For example, Bianchine et al.[14] showed that slow gastric emptying may reduce the clinical effectiveness of levodopa. Age-related changes in GI physiology have caused reduced absorption of substances that are actively transported.[15,16,17] However, apart from the above, there appears to be little evidence to indicate that the absorption efficiency of passively absorbed substances is decreased in healthy aged individuals.[5]

The situation is somewhat different when one considers other factors. The physiological changes that occur in the GI tract with age, however subtle, are likely to increase the susceptibility of drug absorption processes to the influence of other substances. As stated previously, elderly patients tend to take medication with meals for convenience, and the effect of the meal on drug absorption in a somewhat older and less efficient GI system is likely to be greater than in a younger person.

Two other factors must be considered. Diseases of the GI tract tend to be more common among older individuals. Several GI conditions, including achlorhydria, surgery, atrophic gastritis, pyloric stenosis, celiac disease, Crohn's disease, small bowel diverticulosis, regional enteritis, and colitis, have been shown to affect drug absorption.[18] In situations in which absorption is adversely affected, exacerbation of these changes due to other substances would be undesirable. The second factor is the generally greater susceptibility of the older patient to changes in the therapeutic efficacy of a drug. The greater dependency of many elderly patients on chronic therapy, the inevitable concern that may arise from an altered clinical effect, and the reduced ability of the elderly patient to cope with the clinical consequences of altered drug absorption would make this patient population particularly vulnerable to changes in drug absorption due to interactions with food or other substances.

PHYSIOLOGICAL EFFECTS OF FOOD ON THE GASTROINTESTINAL TRACT

Ingestion of food influences GI physiology in terms of motility, secretions, and blood flow.[1,2] Most reports on stomach emptying have utilized liquid or semiliquid meals, and their relevance to the situation with solid meals is uncertain. The presence of liquid food may increase the stomach-emptying rate, presumably by activating stretch receptors in the stomach wall.[19,20] However, the predominant result of food ingestion, particularly solid meals, is to delay stomach emptying as a result of feedback mechanisms by receptors in the proximal small intestine.[2,19] Stomach emptying is delayed by hot meals, by solutions of high viscosity, and also by high-fat, and, to a lesser extent, by high-carbohydrate and high-protein meals.[2]

Since the primary site for absorption of most orally administered drugs is the proximal small intestine, delayed stomach emptying may influence drug absorption to a variable degree. Prolonged residence of basic drugs in the acidic environment of the stomach may increase the fraction that is dissolved when it eventually reaches the small intestine. If the basic drug is unstable in acidic solution, e.g. erythromycin, then delayed stomach emptying may cause drug degradation and reduced availability. Prolonged residence of acidic drugs in the stomach may lead to slower dissolution and reduced availability. On the other hand, if the drug is soluble at acidic pH, absorption from the stomach may increase, as the drug will be in solution in the unionized, readily absorbable form. When drug absorption occurs at a specific site in the intestine, commonly called an "absorption window," delayed stomach emptying may lead to increased absorption by reducing the rate at which the drug passes this site.[21]

Food increases small intestinal motility, and this may accelerate drug dissolution and also decrease the mean free path of drug molecules to the intestinal epithelium, leading to increased absorption. On the other hand, increased intestinal motility may reduce absorption because of increased drug transit rate through the intestine.

Food ingestion leads to increased GI secretion of a number of substances. The most important of these, as far as drug interactions are concerned, are probably the secretion of hydrochloric acid into the stomach and of bile into the duodenum. Increased acid secretion is likely to affect the dissolution and degree of ionization of acidic and basic drugs. Bile secretion is likely to increase the dissolution of lipid-soluble substances.[22,23] Bile may also promote drug absorption by facilitating the dissolution of lipid coatings and waxy matrices in some dosage forms, but it may also reduce absorption efficiency because of bile salt-drug complexation.[24]

The ingestion of food generally causes an increase in splanchnic blood flow, and drug absorption may be influenced by this, depending on the mechanism governing its absorption. Passive drug absorption might be expected to increase with increasing blood flow because of transluminal concentration gradient. If drug absorption is limited by membrane transport phenomena, absorption should not be influenced by blood flow rate. Altered splanchnic blood flow may also affect the absorption of orally dosed drugs that are extensively metabolized in the liver. The extent to which absorption is affected is influenced by the hepatic extraction efficiency. If extraction efficiency is low, then increased splanchnic blood flow may give rise to increased systemic drug availability. However, if increased blood flow is prolonged beyond the drug absorption time, the total area under the blood level/time curve may be unchanged because of the compensating influence of faster overall hepatic metabolism.[25] If hepatic extraction efficiency is high, then altered blood flow should not affect drug availability.[2]

FOOD-DRUG INTERACTIONS

Drug availability may be affected by direct interactions between drug molecules and food components. For example, drugs may chelate with polyvalent metals or may complex with proteins.[26] Food may also act as a mechanical barrier, preventing drug access to the epithelial surface of the GI tract. Food may also indirectly inhibit drug absorption because of digestion by GI secretions.

INFLUENCE OF FLUID VOLUME ON DRUG ABSORPTION

The volume of water that is ingested with a drug may cause a significant change in its absorption. Contrary to earlier suggestions,[27] studies in experimental animals[28,29] and in humans[30,31,32] have indicated that drug absorption increases when the drug is administered in a large fluid volume. This increased absorption appears to be due to the combined effects of accelerated stomach emptying,[1] exposure of dissolved drug molecules to a larger GI surface area, and faster drug dissolution. The stomach tends to contain less water with advancing age, so that administering drugs with larger fluid volumes may be more important in elderly than in young patients.[7]

SPECIFIC FOOD-DRUG INTERACTIONS

Drugs that are most commonly used by elderly patients may be separated into the following categories: (1) anti-infective agents; (2) analgesic and anti-inflammatory agents; (3) antianxiety, sedative, and antidepressant drugs; and (4) cardiac drugs, antihypertensives, and diuretics. In the following sections, known effects of food and fluid volumes on the absorption of some drugs in the above categories will be discussed.

Food can cause drug absorption to be reduced, delayed, increased, or it may have no effect. Which of these occurs is dependent on the drug, the formulation in which it is administered, when it is taken relative to meals, and the type of meal. Given all of these factors, it is not surprising that divergent results of food-drug interactions are often reported for the same compound from different laboratories.

The results presented in this review must therefore be considered in this light, with due cognizance that many reports have been obtained using a single experimental procedure and may not necessarily apply under different conditions.

Anti-infective Agents

The influence of food on the absorption of antimicrobial and antifungal agents has been reviewed.[33] While the results of various studies have fallen into all four categories—i.e., reduced, delayed, unaffected, or increased absorption—the reduced and delayed categories predominate.

Compounds whose absorption may be reduced by the presence of food are shown in Table 3-1. Here, as elsewhere in this review, compounds may appear in more than one category. For example amoxicillin, penicillin V (acid), and pivampicillin appear in Tables 3-1 and 3-3, while various erythromycin products appear in Tables 3-1, 3-2, 3-3, and 3-4. While this may be confusing to the reader, it is unavoidable. In many instances,—e.g., erythromycins—divergent results are predominantly due to different formulations. In other cases, different results may be due to a number of factors, including the conditions employed in particular studies.

Reduced Drug Absorption   Independent studies have shown that circulating levels of penicillin V may be significantly reduced by food, whether the penicillin is administered as the potassium or calcium salt, or as the free acid.[34,35,36] When 150-mg oral doses of penicillin V were given to healthy subjects under fasting and nonfasting conditions, peak antibiotic levels in serum were reduced by 75%, 80%, and 60% for the potassium, calcium, and acid forms, respectively, when they were taken with food.[35] Mean serum antibiotic levels in 45 subjects receiving phenethicillin or penicillin V before, with, and after a standard

Table 3-1. Anti-infective agents whose absorption may be reduced by food

Compound	Reference
Penicillin V (Ca)	34
Penicillin V (acid)	35
Penicillin V (K)	36
Penicillin G	37
Phenethicillin	36,38
Amoxicillin	32
Ampicillin	32,39
Pivampicillin	40,41,42
Nafcillin	43
Cephalexin	44
Tetracycline	45,46,47,48
Oxytetracycline	46
Demethylchlortetracycline	46
Methacycline	48
Isoniazid	49
Rifampin	50
Erythromycin	51,52
Erythromycin stearate	53,54,55,56,57
Slightly Reduced	
Doxycycline	45,48,58

meal are shown in Figure 3-1.[36] Lower serum antibiotic activity because of food is evident for both compounds, but the effect is greater for phenethicillin. Serum antibiotic levels were depressed, compared with the fasting state, even when drugs were taken three hours after a meal.

The systemic availability of ampicillin is reduced by food.[32,39] Figure 3-2 illustrates mean serum ampicillin profiles following administration of ampicillin trihydrate capsules to volunteers under fasting and nonfasting conditions.[32] The overall availability of ampicillin was reduced approximately 50% by each of the test meals examined. The effect of food on amoxicillin absorption is variable, some studies indicating reduction,[32] others showing little effect.[59] The absorption of amoxicillin is also affected by the accompanying fluid volume, circulating levels in fasted subjects being doubled when the drug is taken with 250 ml, compared with 25 ml, of water.[32] For further studies concerning amoxicillin/food interactions, see reference 33.

Pivampicillin, an ampicillin derivative, is often taken with meals to avoid gastric irritation. A number of studies have reported reduced pivampicillin absorption due to food,[40,41,42] but other studies have shown little or no effect (See Table

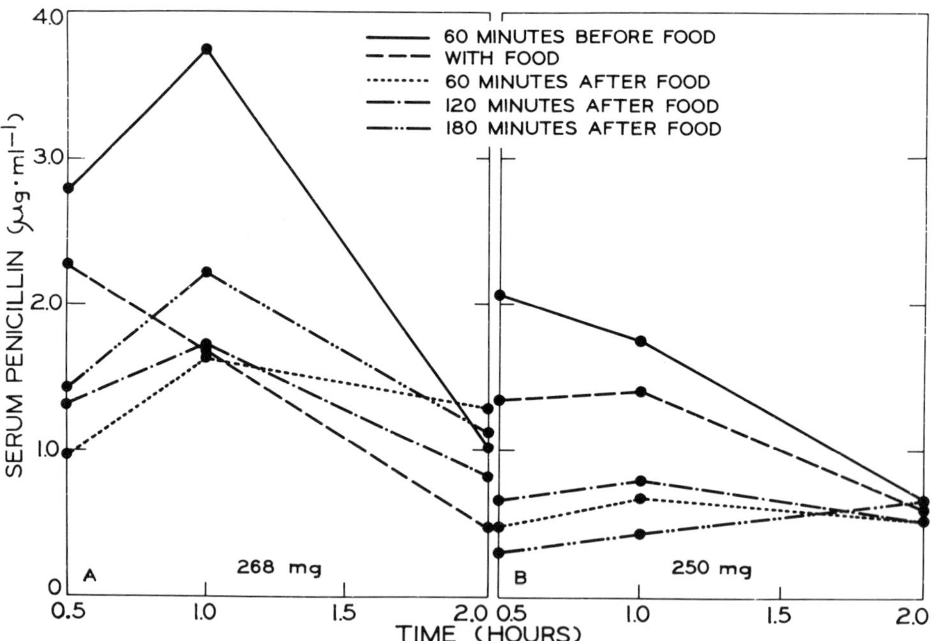

Fig. 3.1. Mean serum antibiotic levels in 45 subjects following oral administration of potassium phenethicillin (A) or penicillin V (B) one hour before, with, one hour after, two hours after, and three hours after a standard meal. With permission of Slack, Inc. from Cronk, BA, Wheatley, WM, Fellers GF, Albright H: The relationship of food intake to the absorption of potassium alpha-phenoxethyl penicillin and potassium phenoxymethyl penicillin from the gastrointestinal tract. Am J Med Sci 240:219, 1960.

3-1). Fernandez et al.[42] reported a 26% reduction in the mean peak serum level and a 46% reduction in the area under the serum curve when pivampicillin was administered with food. Circulating levels of nafcillin are lower, less reproducible, and are achieved more slowly when this antibiotic is given after a meal, compared with the fasting state.[43]

It is well known that the systemic availability of tetracyclines is reduced by a number of substances, including antacids and heavy metal ions. Availability is also affected by food. The relative influence of food on doxycycline and tetracycline availability is illustrated in Figure 3-3.[45] The test meals significantly reduced serum tetracycline levels, but doxycycline levels were reduced to only a minor extent. Doxycycline absorption is also affected less by milk and other dairy products than other tetracyclines.[46]

Peak serum levels of isoniazid were reduced by 70% and overall bioavailability by 40% when this compound was taken after a standard breakfast, compared with the fasting state.[49] As the therapeutic efficacy of isoniazid is related to serum concentrations, this drug should be taken on an empty stomach. There are conflicting reports on the effects of food on rifampin availability, varying from delayed absorption to marked reduction. A recent study showed a 25% reduction in rifampin serum levels and urinary recovery when single 600-mg doses were given after a high-fat breakfast.[50] Despite this finding, serum antibiotic levels still exceeded the minimum inhibitory concentration for Mycobacterium tuberculosis for ten hours after dosing.

The availability of drug from most erythromycin base and erythromycin stea-

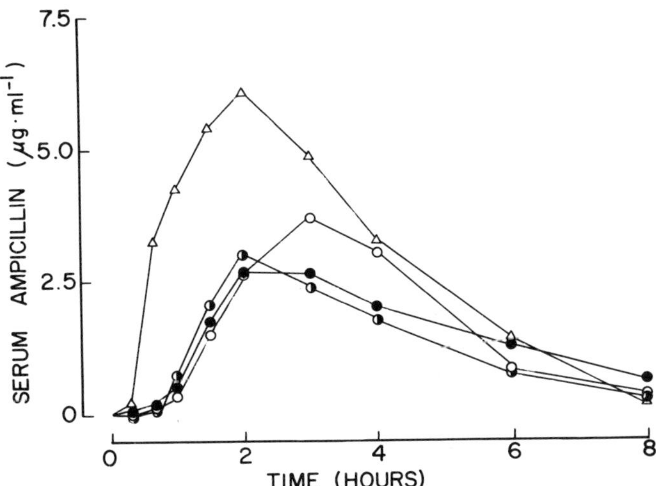

Fig. 3.2.   Mean serum ampicillin levels in six male volunteers following single 500-mg oral doses of ampicillin trihydrate after overnight fast ($\triangle$) and after high-carbohydrate ($\bigcirc$), high-fat ($\bullet$), and high-protein ($\oplus$) meals. Welling PG, Huang H, Koch PA, et al.: Bioavailability of ampicillin and amoxicillin in fasted and nonfasted subjects. J Pharm Sci 66:549, 1977. Reproduced with permission of the copyright owner.

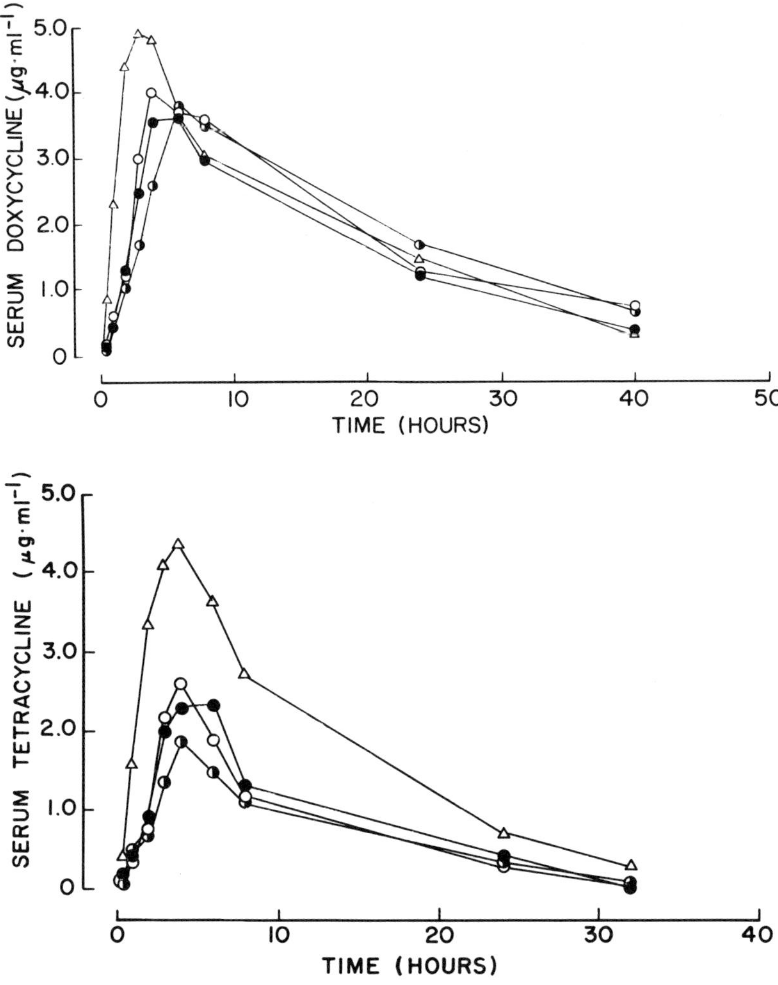

Fig. 3.3.   Mean serum doxycycline (A) and tetracycline (B) levels in six male volunteers following single oral doses of doxycycline hyclate (200 mg) or tetracycline hydrochloride (500 mg) as capsules after overnight fast (A) and after high-carbohydrate (○), high-fat (●), and high-protein (◑) meals. With permission from Welling PG, Koch PA, Lau CC, Craig WA: Bioavailability of tetracycline and doxycycline in fasted and nonfasted subjects. Antimicrob Ag Chemother 11:462, 1977.

rate dosage forms is inhibited by food intake,[52-57] but multiple-dose studies have shown that enteric-coated erythromycin base is influenced less than other formulations.[63] One study has shown that, contrary to the postprandial effect, the systemic availability of erythromycin stearate may significantly increase if it is taken immediately before a meal.[64] Formulation factors may also have influenced the results obtained in that study.

Delayed Drug Absorption   Included in this category are drugs or drug products whose rate of absorption is reduced, while the extent of absorption appears to be unaffected, by the presence of food in the GI tract. Compounds that behave in this way are listed in Table 3-2, and they include most of the oral cephalosporins and sulfonamides. The lack of effect by food on the overall availability of these compounds is probably related, at least in part, to their greater chemical stability in acidic media. In some cases, the results of studies concerning cephalosporin bioavailability have been divergent.[33] For example, Harvengt et al.[65] reported only minor differences in serum levels of cephradine and cephalexin in fasted and nonfasted subjects, while Mischler et al.[66] reported marked delays in cephradine absorption when this compound was taken immediately following a meal. Delayed absorption of oral cephalosporins due to food has also been reported by Glynne et al.[67] in adults and by McCracken et al.[37] in children.

Both of the studies referred to in Table 3-2 indicate that absorption of sulfonamide is delayed by food, but the effects on serum levels may be both compound dependent and formulation dependent. Serum profiles of sulfasymazine, sulfamethoxypyridazine, sulfadimethoxine, sulfisoxazole, and sodium sulfadiazine were decreased as well as being delayed by food. On the other hand, peak levels of sulfanilamide were reduced only slightly, whereas levels from a similar dose of sulfadiazine actually increased.[68,69]

Metronidazole absorption has been studied in healthy volunteers and also in patients with Crohn's disease.[70] Absorption was variable and lower in the patients, but in both groups drug profiles were delayed when metronidazole was taken with food. Delayed, but not reduced, absorption of erythromycin from coated tablets[52] and of erythromycin ethylsuccinate from film-coated tablets[71] has been reported.

Drug Absorption Unaffected   The small number of compounds included in this category are shown in Table 3-3. The lack of effect by food on the absorption of amoxicillin and pivampicillin has been discussed earlier in connection with other studies that have reported reduced absorption of these agents. Circulating levels of spiramycin were similar following a 1.5-gm dose to fasting and nonfasting volunteers, although there was greater variation in the levels among nonfasting individuals.[72] Virtually superimposable serum sulfaisodimidine levels were ob-

Table 3-2. Anti-infective agents whose absorption may be delayed by food

Compound	Reference
Cephalexin	66
Cephradine	65,66
Cefaclor	67
Sulfadimethoxine	68
Sulfamethoxypyridazine	68
Sulfasymazine	68
Sulfisoxazole	68
Sulfanilamide	69
Sulfadiazine	69
Metronidazole	70
Erythromycin	52
Erythromycin ethylsuccinate	71

Table 3-3. Anti-infective agents whose absorption may be unaffected by food

Compound	Reference
Amoxicillin	59
Pivampicillin	60,61,62
Penicillin V (acid)	34
Spiramycin	72
Sulfaisodimidine	73
Erythromycin	51
Erythromycin estolate	74
Erythromycin ethylsuccinate	75

tained when the drug was taken after food and on an empty stomach.[73]

Reports of unaffected absorption of erythromycin and two of its esters[74,75] illustrate the variable results that have been obtained with erythromycin derivatives. Most studies have indicated reduced absorption of erythromycin (Table 3-1, but see reference 63) and increased absorption of erythromycin esters (Table 3-4) in the presence of food.

Increased Drug Absorption Compounds whose absorption may be increased by food are listed in Table 3-4, Although the exact mechanisms that cause altered drug absorption in the presence of food are largely unknown, increased absorption is usually rationalized in terms of increased drug solubility due to the lipids in food, to delayed gastric emptying, or to increased GI secretions. Increased absorption of griseofulvin in the presence of fatty food is an excellent example. Griseofulvin is a highly lipophilic compound, and the presence of fatty food components, delayed stomach emptying, and increased bile secretion all favor increased availability of this compond.[23,76,77] The absorption of griseofulvin appears not to be affected by high-protein or high-carbohydrate meals.[76]

Absorption of nitrofurantoin is increased by food; this absorption may be related to increased dissolution caused by delayed stomach emptying.[78,79] The dramatic effect exerted by food on nitrofurantoin urine levels in one individual is shown in Figure 3-4. In a panel of subjects, mean urinary recovery of nitrofurantoin increased from circa 8% in fasted subjects to 24% when the drug was taken after food.

While the availability of most sulfonamides is delayed or unaffected by food, the absorption of sulfamethoxydiazine appears to increase.[80,81] Although plasma levels were delayed, peak plasma concentrations of sulfamethoxydiazine were increased, and the area under the plasma curve was almost doubled after postprandial doses. Increased availability of the dipeptide alafosfin in the presence of milk,

Table 3-4. Anti-infective agents whose absorption may be increased by food

Compound	Reference
Griseofulvin	76,77
Nitrofurantoin	78,79
Sulfamethoxydiazine	81
Alafosfin	82
Hetacillin	83
Erythromycin estolate	53,75,84
Erythromycin ethylsuccinate	71,75

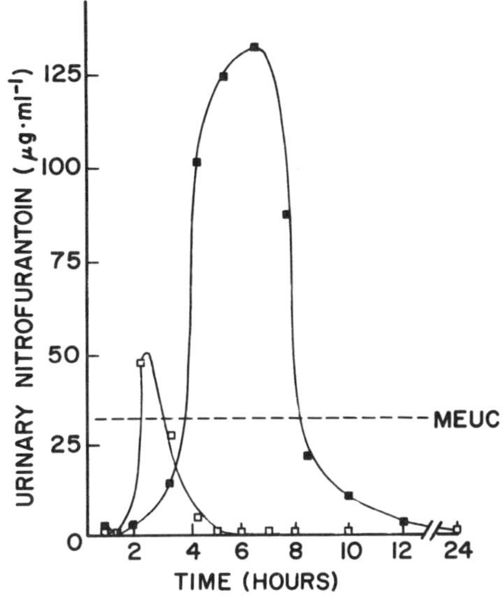

Fig. 3.4. Urinary nitrofurantoin concentrations in one subject following an oral dose of 100 mg microcrystalline nitrofurantoin under fasting (□) and nonfasting (■) conditions. MEUC is the minimum effective urinary concentration agent Enterobacteriaceae (32 mg/1). With permission from Rosenberg HA, Bates TR: The influence of food on nitrofurantoin bioavailability. Clin Pharmacol Ther 20:227, 1976.

and to a lesser extent in the presence of protein, may be related to competitive inhibition for intestinal peptidases, thereby reducing enzymic degradation of alafosfin before absorption from the GI tract.[82] The absorption of hetacillin, the ampicillin precursor, is shown to increase when administered with meals.[83]

The esters of erythromycin, in particular the estolate and the ethylsuccinate esters are less water soluble and more resistant to acid-catalyzed degradation than the free base or its salts. They can consequently be taken in encapsulated and suspension dosage forms. Although there is some divergence among reports of the effects of food on these forms of erythromycin, most studies report either little effect or increased absorption when they are taken after meals.[53,71,75,84] The extent to which circulating levels of total erythromycin (the esterified form plus the free base) may be increased by the presence of food is indicated in Figure 3-5.[75]

Analgesic and Anti-inflammatory Agents

This category of drugs, and also those considered subsequently in this chapter, are heavily prescribed for older patients. It is unfortunate, therefore, that so few food-drug interaction studies have been carried out for these compounds. For most drugs in this and the following categories, the influence of food on absorption and the potential clinical efficacy are not known. Results of some studies concerning analgesic and anti-inflammatory agents are summarized in Table 3-5.

The influence of food, or of changes in accompanying fluid volume, on the absorption and circulating levels of aspirin have been studied using a variety of dosage forms in healthy volunteers.[85,86,91] In one study, 650-mg doses of conventional aspirin tablets were administered with 25 ml or 250 ml of water to healthy fasting volunteers, and also following standardized high-carbohydrate, high-fat, or high-protein solid meals. Mean plasma levels of unchanged aspirin (acetylsalicylate) following these various treatments are shown in Figure 3-6.[85] Mean peak plasma levels of 9 μg/ml and 7 μg/ml were obtained within approximately one-half hour from the 250-ml and 25-ml fasting treatments respectively. Peak acetylsalicylate levels were obtained between one-half hour and two hours following the postprandial doses, and peak plasma levels decreased to circa 4 μg/ml, i.e., a 50% reduction in peak levels due to food. Thus, a reduced accompanying fluid volume caused a decrease in circulating aspirin levels, but not to the same extent as caused by food. Circulating levels of salicylate, a major metabolite of aspirin with anti-pruritic activity, exhibited similar trends to the parent drug, but differences between plasma profiles from the different treatments were not as great.

In a different study, subjects received aspirin in the form of enteric-coated tablets, and also as enteric-coated granules in capsules, after overnight fast and following a standard breakfast.[86] The mean plasma salicylate levels obtained are shown in Figure 3-7. The plasma profiles from the coated tablets were both depressed and delayed in nonfasting subjects, but food had little effect on absorption from the coated granules. This finding probably relates to the more diffuse nature of the granule dosage form and to the greater ease with which granules can pass from the acid region of the stomach to the relatively alkaline proximal small intestine, facilitating faster breakdown of the acid-resistant enteric coating. The absorption of aspirin from a combination tablet, also containing antipyrine and

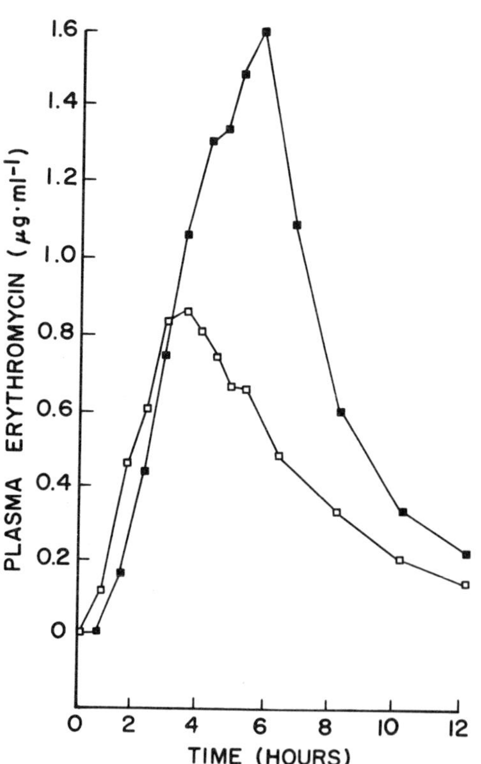

Fig. 3.5. Mean plasma levels of total erythromycin (ester and free base) in 20 subjects following a single 250-mg oral dose of erythromycin estolate as capsules two hours before (□) and one hour after (■) beginning a standard meal. With permission from Bechtol LD, Bessent CT, Perkal MB: The influence of food on the absorption of erythromycin esters and enteric-coated erythromycin in single-dose studies. Curr Ther Res 25:618, 1979.

Table 3-5. Influence of food on the absorption of analgesic and anti-inflammatory agents

Drug	Effect on Absorption	Reference
Aspirin (tablets)	Reduced	85
Aspirin (enteric-coated tablets)	Reduced	86
Acetaminophen	Reduced	87
Aspirin (enteric-coated tablets)	Delayed	86
Alclofenac	Delayed	88
Indoprofen (capsules)	Delayed	89
Indomethacin	Delayed	90
Aspirin (enteric-coated granules)	Unaffected	86
Aspirin (combination tablets)	Unaffected	91
Acetaminophen	Unaffected	87
Indoprofen (tablets)	Unaffected	89

dextropropoxyphene, was unaffected by food,[91] but the absorption of alclofenac was delayed when this drug was administered as a suspension immediately before or 30 minutes after a standard breakfast.[88]

Different effects of food were observed on the absorption of two different dosage forms of indoprofen.[89] Circulating drug levels were delayed when an encapsulated dosage form was given following a standard meal. When indoprofen was given in the form of tablets, the absorption rate was increased slightly, whereas the extent of absorption was unaffected. The authors suggest that the rate of indoprofen absorption from capsules may be limited by gastric emptying time whereas absorption from the tablets may be dependent on tablet disintegration or dissolution rates.[89] Meals that are rich in carbohydrates appear to reduce the availability of acetaminophen, whereas meals that have high-fat or high-protein content have little effect.[87]

Plasma levels of indomethacin were delayed by high-fat, high-protein, and high-carbohydrate meals, relative to the fasting state.[90] The high-carbohydrate meal exhibited the greatest effect, delaying the time of peak plasma concentrations to 2 hours, compared with 1.5 hours from the other test meals and 45 minutes in

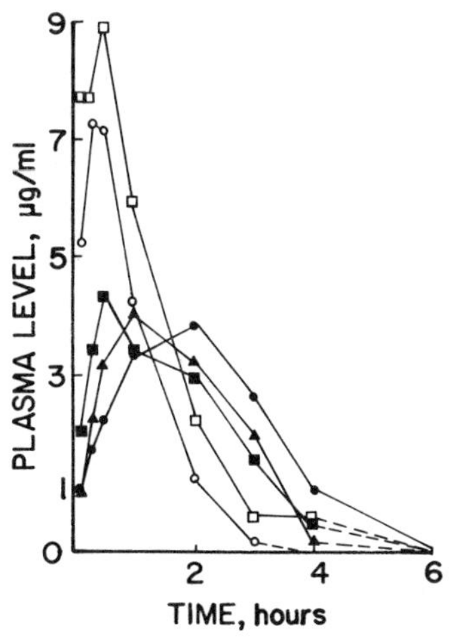

Fig. 3.6. Mean plasma levels of acetylsalicylate in six healthy subjects following single 650-mg oral dose of aspirin in tablets after overnight fast with 250 ml (□) and 25 ml (○) of water, and after high-carbohydrate (●), high-fat (▲), and high protein (■) meals. Koch PA, Schultz CA, Wills RJ, et al.: Influence of food and fluid ingestion on aspirin bioavailability. J Pharm Sci 67, 1533, 1978. Reproduced with permission of the copyright owner.

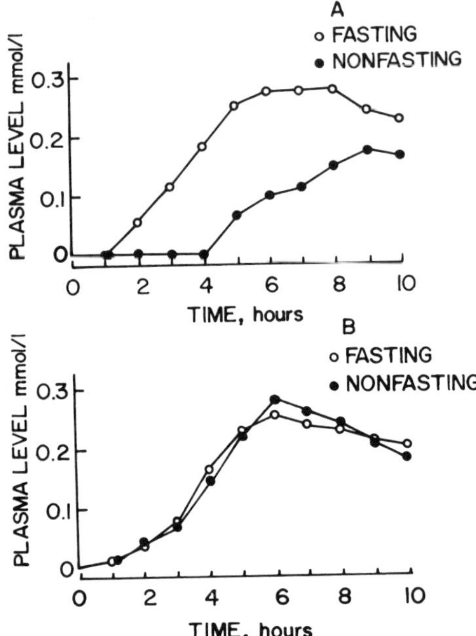

Fig. 3.7. Mean plasma salicylate levels following single 1-gm oral doses of aspirin as enteric-coated tablets (A) and enteric-coated granules in capsules (B), under fasting and nonfasting conditions. With permission from Bogentoft C, Carlsson I, Ekenved G, Magnusson A: Influence of food on the absorption of acetylsalicyclic acid from enteric-coated dosage forms. Eur J Clin Pharmacol 14:351, 1978.

fasting subjects. However, the amount of drug absorbed after 24 hours was similar following all fasting and nonfasting treatments. Administering indomethacin with meals may thus be useful to reduce GI side effects associated with this drug. The mean plasma profiles of indomethacin from the four treatments are shown in Figure 3-8. The absorption of indomethacin and phenylbutazone has been shown to be similar in young and elderly individuals,[92,93] but the effect of food has not been studied in the elderly.

Antianxiety, Sedative, and Antidepressant Drugs

There have been very few studies on the effect of food on the availability of or on the clinical effects of compounds in this category. Among the benzodiazepines, the availability of oxazepam is unaffected by food,[94] whereas diazepam[95,96] and carbamazepine[97] are both increased. In the case of carbamazepine, the overall increase in drug availability due to food in six subjects was not significant, but the increase in the mean peak plasma level from 4.5 μg/ml in fasting individuals to 5.7 μg/ml after postprandial doses was highly significant (p = 0.003). The bioavailability of lorazepam is unaffected by age,[98] but food interactions with this drug appear not to have been studied.

Cardiac Drugs, Antihypertensives and Diuretics

Drugs in this category are listed in Table 3-6. Doses of digoxin have to be carefully adjusted to suit the needs of the patient. While digoxin absorption is not decreased in elderly patients, it is delayed.[99,100] The clearance of digoxin from the body is also lower in the older patient.[100]

While no studies have examined the influence of food on digoxin availability in elderly patients, studies in younger subjects indicate that absorption is delayed after postprandial tablet doses.[104,105] No differences were observed in mean serum digoxin levels between fasting and nonfasting subjects receiving digoxin elixir.[105] Although there was no apparent effect by food on the overall digoxin availability in any of these studies, there was considerable variation among individuals. Individual response should therefore be carefully monitored, not only for patients who may change their digoxin therapy, but also for those who may receive the same dose of medication under different conditions.

Food and fluid volumes have been shown to have variable effects on the availability and circulating levels of some beta adrenergic blocking agents. Plasma levels of atenolol[101] and sotalol[102] are reduced by food, and levels of sotalol are also reduced by concomitant milk or calcium gluconate intake.[102] Large fluid volumes and calcium treatments also reduce the rate of sotalol absorption, but a ferrous sulfate solution has little effect. Food does not influence the absorption of oxprenolol, whether it is taken as conventional or slow-release tablets.[106]

Contrary to the above results, food causes a marked increase in circulating levels of propranolol, metoprolol,[109] and labetalol.[110] Typical serum levels of

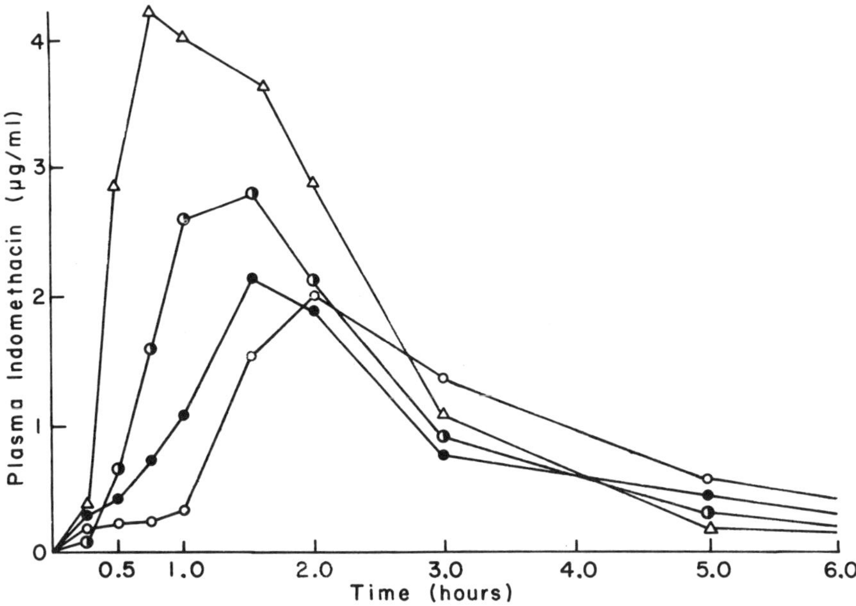

Fig. 3.8. Mean plasma indomethacin levels following single 100-mg oral doses of indomethacin after overnight fast ($\triangle$) and after high-carbohydrate ($\bigcirc$), high-fat ($\bullet$), and high-protein ($\boldsymbol{\varodot}$) meals. With permission from Wallusch WW, Nowak H, Leopold G, Netter KJ: Comparative bioavailability: Influence of various diets on the bioavailability of indomethacin. Int J Clin Pharmacol 16:40, 1978.

Table 3-6. Influence of food on the absorption of cardiac drugs, antihypertensives, and diuretics

Drug	Effect on Absorption	Reference
Atenolol	Reduced	101
Sotalol	Reduced	102
Hydrochlorothiazide	Reduced	103
Digoxin (tablets)	Delayed	104,105
Digoxin (elixir)	Unaffected	105
Oxprenolol	Unaffected	106
Bendroflumethiazide	Unaffected	107
Canrenone	Increased	108
Propranolol	Increased	109
Metoprolol	Increased	110
Labetalol	Increased	110
Hydralazine	Increased	111
Chlorothiazide	Increased	112

propranolol and metoprolol in fasting and nonfasting subjects are shown in Figure 3-9. It is not clear why food has such different effects on the absorption of these compounds. It is interesting, however, that the compounds whose absorption is increased by food—metoprolol, propranolol, and labetalol—are extensively metabolized by the liver and undergo first-pass hepatic metabolism. Sotalol and atenolol on the other hand, whose absorption is inhibited by food, are not significantly metabolized. Increased availability of the extensively metabolized compounds may therefore be related to changes in splanchnic blood flow following food intake. A possible mechanism whereby this may occur has been suggested by McLean et al.[25] The apparent lack of effect by food on oxprenolol systemic availability may be due to a combination of the opposing effects of reduced first-pass metabolism and of reduced absorption due to interactions with meal components in the GI tract.[25]

Variable effects of food have also been observed with the thiazide diuretics, although the possible rationales for these are different from those proposed for the beta-blocking agents. The absorption of bendroflumethiazide is unaffected, and that of hydrochlorothiazide is decreased to a small but significant extent when these compounds are taken after meals.[103,107] A previous study using somewhat different conditions has reported a slight increase in hydrochlorothiazide absorption following postprandial doses, but the increases were not considered to be clinically significant.[113] Contrary to these observations, the systemic availability of the closely related compound chlorothiazide was doubled when administered following a standard meal, compared with overnight fast. Absorption was also increased when the drug was accompanied by a large water volume, but the differences in availability resulting from the large and small fluid volumes were not statistically significant.[112] The cumulative percentage urinary recovery of unchanged chlorothiazide from the different treatments is shown in Figure 3-10.

The different effects exerted by food on the availability of the thiazide diuretics may be rationalized in terms of their relative absorption efficiencies. Bendroflumethiazide and hydrochlorothiazide are efficiently absorbed from the GI tract, and food is unlikely to markedly increase their absorption further. Chlorothiazide, on the other hand, is absorbed with lower efficiency and exhibits a marked "absorption window" effect. A reduction in gastric emptying rate due to food is likely to decrease the rate and concentration at which chlorothiazide passes the absorption site, leading to more efficient absorption.[112]

Plasma levels of canrenone[108] (metabolite of spironolactone) and hydralazine[111] are enhanced by concomitant food intake.

SUMMARY AND CONCLUSIONS

The proportion of the population that may be considered elderly is increasing, and will continue to do so as life expectancy increases. It is therefore important to understand how the elderly patient handles administered drugs, and the clinical consequences of drug interactions with other substances.

As indicated earlier in this chapter, there is little evidence that a healthy older patient will absorb orally administered drugs differently from a younger individual. However with some agents—for example, digoxin—slower absorption, together with drug distribution changes with age, can affect patient response. Physiological changes do occur in the aging GI tract, and these may give rise to greater patient susceptibility to interactions that influence drug absorption. The elderly patient suffers from the additional disadvantages of being susceptible to an

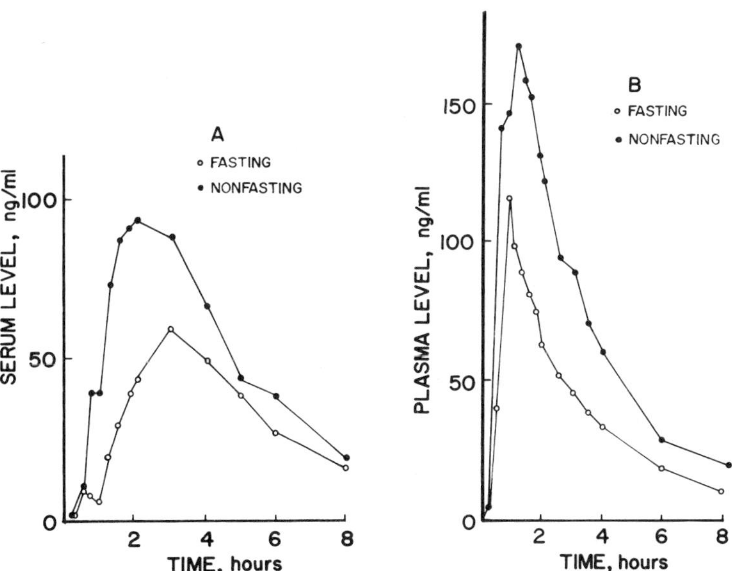

Fig. 3.9.   Serum propranolol (A) and plama metroprolol (B) levels in two subjects following single doses of 80 mg propranolol or 100 mg metoprolol under fasting and nonfasting conditions. With permission from Melander A, Danielson K, Scherstén B, Wahlin E: Enhancement of the bioavailability of propranolol and metoprolol by food. Clin Pharmacol Ther 22:108, 1977.

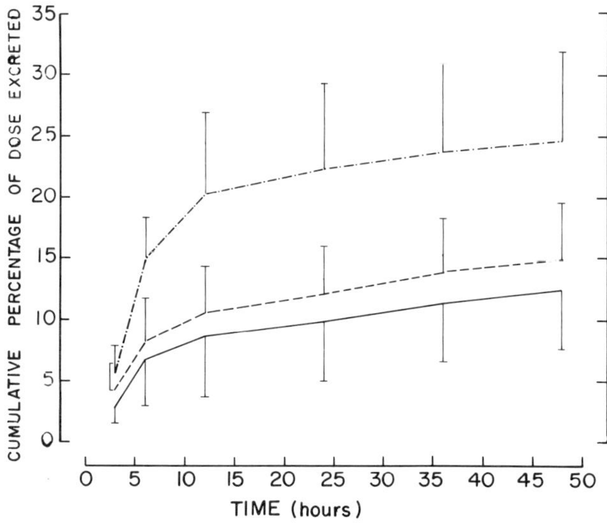

Fig. 3.10. Mean cumulative percentage of 500-mg chlorothiazide dose recovered in urine of nine subjects receiving the drug after overnight fast with 250 ml of water (---) or 25 ml of water (—), and following a standard breakfast ($-\cdot-\cdot$). Welling PG, Barbhaiya RH: Influence of food and fluid volume on chlorothiazide bioavailability: Comparison of plasma and urinary excretion methods. J Pharm Sci 71:32, 1982. Reproduced with permission of the copyright owner.

increasing number of disease conditions that influence drug absorption and, in some cases, a potentially reduced ability to cope with clinical changes brought about by altered drug absorption.

Thus, it is important that we understand the various factors influencing drug efficacy in the elderly patient. Despite this fact, practically all of the present information regarding food-drug interactions affecting absorption has been generated from young, healthy, individuals. While it is likely that many of the types of interactions observed in younger volunteers will occur also in elderly patients, it is more likely that the effects will be greater in the elderly, and will be of greater clinical significance.

The four categories of drugs that were discussed in this review were chosen to represent those compounds heavily prescribed in elderly patients. Many other categories of drugs have not been considered. Also, only sufficient examples within the selected categories were used to illustrate the types of interactions that may occur. More detailed coverage of the many reported food-drug interactions is provided in previous reviews.[1,2,3,33]

It is clear from the examples presented in this chapter that food can cause drug absorption to be reduced, delayed, or increased, or it may be without effect. Which of these occurs is dependent on many factors including the drug and its dosage form, the type of meal, and the fluid volume ingested. Clearly, for optimal absorption, some compounds, including the cephalosporins, tetracyclines, and penicillins should be taken on an empty stomach. Others, including chlorothiazide, the esters of erythromycin, nitrofurantoin, and some beta-blocking agents, appear to be more efficacious when taken after meals. For some drug products, e.g. theophylline,[114] cimetidine,[115] chlorpropamide, and tolbutamide,[116] it is not important from a bioavailability standpoint when they are taken with respect to food.

Of all the food-drug interaction studies, the majority have shown that food either adversely affects or only slightly modifies drug absorption. It is reasonable to suggest, then, that, with the exception of instances in which food has been shown to increase absorption and drugs that cause GI irritation, drugs should be given on an empty stomach.

The paucity of information regarding drug interactions affecting absorption in elderly patients requires that dosing guidelines that have been established in younger patients be used for this population. This unsatisfactory situation will hopefully be rectified as more information becomes available on drug interactions and their clinical consequences in the elderly.

REFERENCES

1. Welling PG: Influence of food and diet on gastrointestinal drug absorption. J Pharmacokin Biopharm 5:291, 1977.
2. Toothaker RD, Welling PG: The effect of food on drug bioavailability. Ann Rev Pharmacol Toxicol 20:173, 1980.
3. Melander A: Influence of food on the bioavailability of drugs. Clin Pharmacokin 3:337, 1978.
4. Geokas MC, Haverback BJ: The aging GI tract. Am J Surg 117:881, 1969.
5. Israili ZH, Wenger J: Aging, gastrointestinal disease and response to drugs. In Jarvik LF, Greenblatt DJ, Harman D (eds): Clinical Pharmacology and the Aged Patient. New York, Raven Press, 1981.
6. Exton-Smith AN: Clinical manifestations. In: Exton-Smith AN, Evans JG (eds): Care of the Elderly. London, Academic Press, 1977, pp 41–53.
7. Lamy PP: Misuse and abuse of drugs by elderly, another view. Am Pharm 20:14–17, 1980.
8. Fikry ME: Gastric secretory functions in the aged. Gerontol Clin 7:216, 1965.
9. Dosherholmen A, Ripley D, Chang S, Silvis SE: Influence of age and stomach functions on serum vitamin B_{12} concentration. Scand J Gastroenterol 12:313, 1977.
10. Blackman AH, Lambert DL, Thayer WR, Martin HF: Computed normal values for peak acid output based on age, sex and body weight. Am J Dig Dis 5:783, 1970.
11. Warren PM, Pepperman MA, Montgomery RD: Age changes in small intestinal mucosa. Lancet 2:849, 1978.
12. Cline WS, Lorenzsonn V, Benz L, et al.: The effects of sodium ricinoleate on small intestinal function and structure. J Clin Invest 58:380, 1976.
13. Meisel JL. Bergman D, Graney D, et al.: Human rectal mucosa: Proctoscopic and morphological changes caused by laxatives. Gastroenterol 72:1274, 1977.
14. Bianchine JR, Calimlim LR, Morgan JP, et al.: Metabolism and absorption of 1-3, 4-dihydroxy-phenylalanine in patients with Parkinson's disease. Ann NY Acad Sci 170:126, 1971.
15. Bender AD: Effect of age on intestinal absorption. J Am Geriat Soc 16:1331, 1968.
16. Meyer J, Sorter H, Oliver J, Necheles H: Studies in old age. Intestinal absorption in old

age. Gastroenterol 1:876, 1943.

17. Sapp OL, Seasions JT, Rose JW: Effect of aging on intestinal absorption of sugars. Clin Res 12:31, 1964.

18. Parsons RL: Drug absorption in gastrointestinal disease with particular reference to malabsorption syndromes. Clin Pharmacokin 2:45, 1977.

19. Hunt JN, Knox MT: Regulation of gastric emptying. In Code CF, Heidel W (eds): Handbook of Physiology. Alimentary Canal. Baltimore, Williams & Wilkins, 1968.

20. Hunt JN, Spurrell WR: The pattern of emptying of the human stomach. J Physiol 113:157, 1951.

21. Levy G, Jusko WJ: Factors affecting the absorption of riboflavin in man. J Pharm Sci 55:285, 1966.

22. Crounse RG: Human pharmacology of griseofulvin: The effect of fat intake on gastrointestinal absorption. J Invest Dermatol 37:529, 1961.

23. Bates TR, Gibaldi M, Kanig JL: Solubilizing properties of bile salt solutions. 2. Effect of inorganic electrolyte, lipids, and a mixed bile salt system on solubilization of glutethimide, griseofulvin, and hexestrol. J Pharm Sci 55:901, 1966.

24. Bates TR, Gibaldi M: Gastrointestinal absorption of drugs. In Swarbrick J (ed): Current Concepts in the Pharmaceutical Sciences: Biopharmaceutics, Philadelphia, Lea and Febiger, 1970, pp 57–99.

25. McLean AJ, McNamara PJ, du Souich P, et al.: Food, splanchnic blood flow, and bioavailability of drugs subject to first-pass metabolism. Clin Pharmacol Ther 24:5, 1978.

26. Kohn KW: Mediation of divalent metal ions in the binding of tetracycline to macromolecules. Nature 191:1156, 1961.

27. Fingl E, Woodbury DM: General principles. In Goodman LS, Gilman A (eds): The Pharmacological Basis of Therapeutics. Macmillan, New York, 1975, pp 1–46.

28. Borowitz JL, Moore PF, Yim GKW, Miya TS: Mechanism of enhanced drug effects produced by dilution of the oral dose. Toxicol Appl Pharmacol 19:164, 1971.

29. Ferguson HC: Dilution of dose and acute oral toxicity. Toxicol Appl Pharmacol 4:759, 1962.

30. Welling PG, Huang H, Hewitt PF, Lyons LL: Bioavailability of erythromycin stearate. J Pharm Sci 67:764, 1978

31. Welling PG: How food and fluid affect drug absorption. Postgrad Med 62:73, 1977.

32. Welling PG, Huang H, Koch, PA, et al.: Bioavailability of ampicillin and amoxicillin in fasted and nonfasted subjects. J Pharm Sci 66:549, 1977.

33. Welling PG, Tse FLS: The influence of food on the absorption of antimicrobial agents. J Antimicrob Chemother 9:7, 1982.

34. Peck FB Jr, Griffith RS: Comparative clinical studies of potassium penicillin V with acid penicillin V. Antibiot Ann 1957:1004, 1958.

35. Berlin H, Brante G: Studies on oral utilization of penicillin V. Antibiot Ann 1958:149, 1959.

36. Cronk GA, Wheatley WB, Fellers GF, Albright H: The relationship of food intake to the absorption of potassium alpha-phenoxyethyl penicillin and potassium phenoxymethyl penicillin from the gastrointestinal tract. Am J Med Sci 240:219, 1960.

37. McCracken GH Jr, Ginsburg CM, Clahsen JC, Thomas ML: Pharmacologic evaluation of orally administered antibiotics in infants and children: Effects of feeding on bioavailability. Pediatrics 62:738, 1978.

38. McCarthy CG, Finland M: Absorption and excretion of four penicillins; penicillin G, penicillin V, phenethicillin, and phenylmercaptomethyl penicillin, New Eng J Med 263, 315, 1960.

39. Neu HC: Antimicrobial activity and human pharmacology of amoxicillin. J Infect Dis 129 (suppl):S123, 1974.
40. Bergan T: Pivampicillin (pondocillin): A new alternative to ampicillin. Tidsskrift for den Norske Laegeforening 92:503, 1972.
41. Magni L, Sjovall J: Absorption of ampicillin and pivampicillin in relation to food intake. Farmaceutisk Tidende 32:645, 1972.
42. Fernandez CA, Menezes JP, Ximenes J: The effect of food on the absorption of pivampicillin and a comparison with the absorption of ampicillin potassium. J Int Med Res 1:530, 1973.
43. Watanakunakorn C: Absorption of orally administered nafcillin in normal healthy volunteers. Antimicrob Ag Chemother 11:1007, 1977.
44. Meyers BR, Kaplan K, Weinstein L: Cephalexin, microbiological effect and pharmacologic parameters in man. Clin Pharmacol Ther 10:810, 1969.
45. Welling PG, Koch PA, Lau CC, Craig WA: Bioavailability of tetracycline and doxycycline in fasted and nonfasted subjects. Antimicrob Ag Chemother 11:462, 1977.
46. Neuvonen P, Mattila M, Gothini G, Hackman R: Interference of iron and milk with absorption of tetracycline. Scand J Clin Lab Invest 27(116):76, 1971.
47. Poieger H, Schlatter C: Compensation of dietary induced reduction of tetracycline absorption by simultaneous administration of EDTA. Eur J Clin Pharmacol 14:129, 1978.
48. Kirby WMM, Roberts CE, Burdick RE: Comparison of two new tetracyclines with tetracycline and demethylchlortetracycline. Antimicrob Ag Chemother 1961:286, 1962.
49. Melander A, Danielson K, Hansen A, et al.: Reduction of isoniazid bioavailability in normal men by concomitant intake of food. Acta Med Scand 200:93, 1976.
50. Siegler DI, Bryant M, Burley DM, et al.: Effect of meals on rifampicin absorption. Lancet 17:197, 1974.
51. Smith JW, Dyke RW, Griffith RS: Absorption following oral administration of erythromycin. JAMA 151:805, 1953.
52. Josselyn LE, Sylvester JC: Absorption of erythromycin. Antibiot Chemother 3:63, 1952.
53. Welling PG, Elliott RL, Pitterle ME, et al.: Plasma levels following single and repeated doses of erythromycin estolate and erythromycin stearate. J Pharm Sci 68:150, 1979.
54. Mäntylä A, Ailio A, Allonen H, Kanto J: Bioavailability and effect of food on the gastrointestinal absorption of two erythromycin derivatives. Ann Clin Res 10:258, 1978.
55. Hirsh HA, Finland M: Effect of food on the absorption of erythromycin propionate, erythromycin stearate and triacetyloleadomycin. Am J Med Sci 237:693, 1959.
56. Welling PG, Huang H, Hewitt PF, Lyons LL: Bioavailability of erythromycin stearate: Influence of food and fluid volume. J Pharm Sci 67:764, 1978.
57. Rutland J, Berend N, Marlin GE: The influence of food on the bioavailability of new formulations of erythromycin stearate and base. Brit J Clin Pharacol 8:343, 1979.
58. Rosenblatt JE, Barrett JE, Brodie JL, Kirby WMM: Comparison of in vitro activity and clinical pharmacology of doxycycline with other tetracyclines. Antimicrob Ag Chemother 1966:134, 1967.
59. Eshelman FM, Spyker DA: Pharmacokinetics of amoxicillin and ampicillin: Crossover study of the effect of food. Antimicrob Ag Chemother 14:539, 1978.
60. Foltz EL, West JW, Breslow IH, Wallick H: Clinical pharmacology of pivampicillin. Antimicrob Ag Chemother 1970:442, 1971.
61. Jordan CM, de Maine J, Kirby W: Clinical pharmacology of pivampicillin as compared with ampicillin, Antimicrob Ag Chemother 1970:438–441, 1971.

62. Roholt K, Nielsen B, Kristensen E: Clinical pharmacology of pivampicillin, Antimicrob Ag Chemother 6:563, 1974.

63. DiSanto AR, Chodos DJ: Influence of study design in assessing food effects on absorption of erythromycin base and erythromycin stearate. Antimicrob Ag Chemother 20:190, 1981.

64. Malmborg AS: Effect of food on absorption of erythromycin: A study of two derivatives, the stearate and the base. J Antimicrob Chemother 5:591, 1979.

65. Harvengt C, de Schepper P, Lamy F, Hansen J: Cephradine absorption and excretion in fasting and nonfasting volunteers. J Clin Pharmacol 13:36, 1973.

66. Mischler TW, Sugermann AA, Willard DA, et al.: Influence of probenecid and food on the bioavailability of cephradine in normal male subjects. J Clin Pharmacol 14:604, 1974.

67. Glynne A, Goulbourn RA, Ryden R: A human pharmacology of cefaclor. J Antimicrob Chemother 4:343, 1978.

68. MacDonald H, Place VA, Falk H, Darken MA: Effect of food on absorption of sulfonamides in man. Chemotherapia 12:282, 1967.

69. Peterson OL, Finland M, Ballou AN: The effect of food and alkali on the absorption and excretion of sulfonamide drugs after oral and duodenal administration. Am J Med Sci 204:581, 1942.

70. Melander A, Kahlmeter G, Kamme C, Ursing B: Bioavailability of metronidazole in fasting and nonfasting healthy subjects and in patients with Crohn's disease. Eur J Clin Pharmacol 12:69, 1977.

71. Thomson PJ, Burgess KR, Marlin GE: Influence of food on absorption of erythromycin ethylsuccinate. Antimicrob Ag Chemother 18:829, 1980.

72. Kamme C, Kahlmeter G, Melander A: Evaluation of spiramycin as a therapeutic agent for elimination of nasopharyngeal pathogens. Scand J Infect Dis 10:135, 1978.

73. Melander A, Wåhlin E, Danielson K, Rerup C: On the influence of concomitant food intake on sulfonamide bioavailability. Acta Med Scand 200:497, 1976.

74. Griffith RS, Joiner M, Kottlowski H: Comparison of antibacterial activity in the sera of subjects ingesting propionyl erythromycin lauryl sulfate and erythromycin ethyl carbonate. Antimicrob Med Clin Ther 7:320, 1960.

75. Bechtol LD, Bessent C, Perkal MB: The influence of food on the absorption of erythromycin esters and enteric-coated erythromycin in single-dose studies. Curr Ther Res 25:618, 1979.

76. Crounse RG: Human pharmacology of griseofulvin: The effect of food intake on gastrointestinal absorption. J Invest Dermatol 37:529, 1961.

77. Kabasakalian P, Katz M, Rosenkrantz B, Townley E: Parameters affecting absorption of griseofulvin using urinary metabolite excretion data. J Pharm Sci 59:595, 1970.

78. Bates TR, Sequeira JA, Tembo AV: Effect of food on nitrofurantoin absorption. Clin Pharmacol Ther 16:63, 1974.

79. Rosenberg HA, Bates TR: The influence of food on nitrofurantoin bioavailability. Clin Pharmacol Ther 20:227, 1976.

80. Kaumeier S: The effect of the composition of food on the absorption of sulfameter. Int J Clin Pharmacol 17:260, 1979.

81. Kaumeier S, Kisslinger E, Neiss A: The effect of gastrointestinal filling on the absorption of sulphamethoxydiazine. Int J Clin Pharmacol 17:412, 1979.

82. Welling PG, Kendall MF, Dean S, et al.: Effect of food on the bioavailability of alafosfalin, a new antibacterial agent. J Antimicrob Chemother 6:373, 1980.

83. Jusko WJ, Lewis GP: Comparison of ampicillin and hetacillin pharmacokinetics in man. J Pharm Sci 62:69, 1973.

84. Abbott Laboratories, North Chicago, Illinois: Bioavailability data: Studies 73–190 and 75–103, 1976.

85. Koch PA, Schultz CA, Wills RJ, et al.: Influence of food and fluid ingestion on aspirin bioavailability. J Pharm Sci 67:1533, 1978.

86. Bogentoft C, Carlsson I, Ekenved G, Magnusson A: Influence of food on the absorption of acetylsalicyclic acid from enteric-coated dosage forms. Eur J Clin Pharmacol 14:351, 1978.

87. Jaffe J, Coliazzi JL, Barry H: Effects of dietary components on gastrointestinal absorption of acetaminophen tablets in man. J Pharm Sci 60:1646, 1971.

88. Sennello LT, Sonders RC, Friedman N: Effect of food on kinetics of the nonsteroidal antiinflammative alclofenac. Clin Pharmacol Ther 23:414, 1978.

89. Tamassia V, Corvi G, Mora E, et al.: Effect of food on absorption of indoprofen administered orally to man in two dosage forms. Int J Clin Pharmacol 15:389, 1977.

90. Wallusch WW, Nowak H, Leopold G, Netter KJ: Comparative bioavailability: Influence of various diets on the bioavailability of indomethacin. Int J Clin Pharmacol 16:40, 1978.

91. Melander A, Berlin-Wåhlin A, Bodin NO, et al.: Bioavailability of d-propoxyphene, acetylsalicyclic acid and phenazone in a combination tablet (Doleron®): Interindividual variation and influence of food intake. Acta Med Scand 202:119, 1977.

92. Trager A, Kunze M, Stein G, Ankermann H: Zür Pharmakokinetik von Indomethacin bei alten Menchen. Z Alternforsch 27:151, 1973.

93. Triggs EJ, Nation RL, Long A, Ashley JJ: Pharmacokinetics in the elderly. Eur J Clin Pharmacol 8:55, 1975.

94. Melander A, Danielson K, Vessman J, Wåhlin E: Bioavailability of oxazepam: Absence of influence of food intake. Acta Pharmacol Toxicol 40:584, 1977.

95. Greenblatt DJ, Allen MD, MacLaughlin DS, et al.: Diazepam absorption: Effect of antacids and food. Clin Pharmacol Ther 24:600, 1978.

96. Linnoila M, Kortilla K, Mattila MJ: Effect of food and repeated injections on serum diazepam levels. Acta Pharmacol Toxicol 36:181, 1975.

97. Levy RH, Pitlick WH, Troupin AS, et al.: Pharmacokinetics of carbamazepine in normal man. Clin Pharmacol Ther 17:657, 1975.

98. Greenblatt DJ, Allen MD, Locniskar A, et al.: Lorazepam kinetics in the elderly. Clin Pharmacol Ther 26:103, 1979.

99. Chavez A, Balant L, Simonin P, Fabre J: Influence de l'âge sur la digoxinémie et la digitalisation. Schweiz Med Wochenschr 104:1823, 1974.

100. Cusak B, Horgan J, Kelly JG, et al.: Pharmacokinetics of digoxin in the elderly. Br J Clin Pharmacol 6:439P, 1978.

101. Melander A, Stenberg P, Liedholm H, et al.: Food-induced reduction in bioavailability of atenolol. Eur J Clin Pharmacol 16:327, 1979.

102. Kahela P, Antilla M, Tikkanen R, Sundquist H: Effect of food and fluid volume on the bioavailability of sotalol. Acta Pharmacol Toxicol 44:7, 1979.

103. Barbhaiya RH, Craig WA, Corrick-West HP, Welling PG: Pharmacokinetics of hydrochlorothiazide in fasted and nonfasted subjects: A comparison of plasma level and urinary excretion methods. J Pharm Sci 71:245, 1982.

104. Johnson BF, O'Grady J, Sabey GA, Bye C; Effect of a standard breakfast on digoxin absorption in normal subjects. Clin Pharmacol Ther 23:315, 1978.

105. Greenblatt DJ, Duhme DW, Koch-Weser J, Smith TW: Bioavailability of digoxin tablets and elixir in the fasting and postprandial states. Clin Pharmacol Ther 16:444, 1974.

106. Dawes CP, Kendall MJ, Welling PG: Bioavailability of conventional and slow-release

oxprenolol in fasted and nonfasted individuals. Br J Clin Pharmacol 7:299, 1979.
107. Beerman B, Groschinsky-Grind M, Lindstrom B: Effect of food on the bioavailability of bendroflumethiazide. Acta Med Scand 204:291, 1978.
108. Melander A, Danielson K, Scherstén B, et al.: Enhancement by food of canrenone bioavailability from spironolactone. Clin Pharmacol Ther 22:100, 1977.
109. Melander A, Danielson K, Scherstén B, Wåhlin E: Enhancement of the bioavailability of propranolol and metoprolol by food. Clin Pharmacol Ther 22:108, 1977.
110. Mäntylä R, Allonen H, Kanto J, et al.: Effect of food on the bioavailability of labetalol. Brit J Clin Pharmacol 9:435, 1980.
111. Melander A, Danielson K, Hanson A, et al.: Enhancement of hydralazine bioavailability by food. Clin Pharmacol Ther 22:104, 1977.
112. Welling PG, Barbhaiya RH: Influence of food and fluid volume on chlorothiazide bioavailability: Comparison of plasma and urinary excretion methods. J Pharm Sci 71:32, 1982.
113. Beerman B, Groschinsky-Grind M: Gastrointestinal absorption of hydrochlorothiazide enhanced by concomitant intake of food. Eur J Clin Pharmacol 13:125, 1978.
114. Welling PG, Lyons LL, Craig WA, Trochta GS: Influence of diet and fluid on bioavailability of theophylline. Clin Pharmacol Ther 17:475, 1975.
115. Bodemar G, Norlander B, Fransson L, Walan A: The absorption of cimetidine before and during maintenance treatment with cimetidine and the influence of a meal on the absorption of cimetidine: Studies in patients with peptic ulcer disease. Br J Clin Pharmacol 7:23, 1979.
116. Sartor G, Melander A, Scherstén B, Wåhlin-Boll E: Influence of food and age on the single dose kinetics and effects of tolbutamide and chloropropamide. Eur J Clin Pharmacol 17:285, 1980.

4 | Nutritional Status and Drug Disposition in the Elderly

Barry Cusack
Michael J. Denham

In a given individual, pharmacological effect depends on the amount of drug that reaches the site of action and on the sensitivity of that person to the drug. Handling of drugs by the body (i.e., absorption, distribution, metabolism, and excretion) is termed *drug disposition,* or *pharmacokinetics.* Pharmacokinetics determines the amount of drug that reaches the site of action. Many factors can affect pharmacokinetics and are of importance since they may change pharmacological response. It is now known that both aging and malnutrition are among such factors, and their effect on pharmacokinetics shall be discussed in some detail in this chapter.

There are many reasons for the rapidly expanding interest in the research of drug kinetics in old age. It has been known for some time that aging is associated with physiological changes that might alter drug disposition. The elderly (those over 65 years) form an increasing proportion of the population of Western nations, their percentage rising in Great Britain from approximately 4% at the turn of the century to over 12% by the year 1961.[1] A similar demographic shift has occurred in the United States.[2] Because the elderly suffer from a high incidence of acute and chronic disease,[3] drug consumption by this group is disproportionately high, accounting in 1976 for 25% of the national total in the United States.[45] Some,[4-6] but not all,[7] reports suggest that adverse drug reactions are more common in old age, possibly because of polypharmacy, altered pharmacokinetics, and altered sensitivity. The effect of aging on pharmacokinetics has now been widely studied and is the subject of many good reviews.[8-12]

Malnutrition is one of the commonest disorders in humans, especially in under-developed regions, where it affects all age groups. Suggestions have been made that malnutrition may be relatively common among the elderly, compared with other age groups, in developed countries.[13] Malnutrition produces changes in physiology and biochemical functions that may alter kinetics, and this relationship in animals and humans is being increasingly examined.[14]

Despite the fact that environmental factors are considered to influence apparent age changes in drug disposition, little attention has been directed toward the role of malnutrition as one such factor. In this review it is proposed to outline the mechanisms and clinical importance of altered drug disposition in old age and malnutrition, and to indicate the possible effect of poor diet on drug disposition in old age.

PHARMACOKINETICS

Pharmacokinetics mathematically describes the way in which drugs are disposed by the body determining the availability of free drug at the site of action. A brief and simple description of pharmacokinetics is germane to the discussion in this chapter. Some excellent short reviews of the subject are available for more detailed explanation.[15,16]

After absorption, each drug distributes throughout a certain space in the body (including site of action). At the same time, elimination of the drug begins by biotransformation (metabolism) and/or renal excretion. The kinetic fate of a drug depends partly on the physicochemical properties of the drug, and also on physiological characteristics of the individual.

Drug distribution can usually be adequately described as occurring in a single compartment or space, so that the larger the compartment, the lower the plasma drug concentration. Only free drug is available for distribution or elimination, and extensive binding of drugs to plasma proteins can limit these processes. The extent of distribution is termed the *apparent volume of distribution* (Vd) and is expressed in liters (l). Fat-soluble drugs distribute mainly into fatty tissues (including the brain). They cross membranes easily and thus distribute widely (mainly into fatty tissues).

Renal elimination of fat-soluble drugs is very limited since, after glomerular filtration, they are reabsorbed from the kidney tubules. Such drugs are metabolized, principally in the liver, into more polar, water-soluble compounds, which can then be excreted by the kidneys.

Metabolism is chiefly catalyzed by a microsomal mixed-function oxidase (MFO) enzyme system located on the smooth endoplasmic reticulum of the hepatocyte. Principal components of this complex include cytochrome P-450, phosphatidylcholine, flavoprotein reductase; the system also requires NADPH and oxygen.

Substrate molecules are made more hydrophilic by this system by the exposure or creation of polar radicals. Most xenobiotic compounds and many endogenous substrates (e.g., steroids) are metabolized by this system. Some drugs are metabolized by nonmicrosomal enzymes, usually by addition of a polar radical (e.g., acetylation).

Rate of drug metabolism is related to the activity of the relevant enzyme system.

Table 4-1. Pathophysiological Changes in Malnutrition

Decrease	Increase
Body fat[20,21]	Total body water[20,26]
Serum albumin[22]	
Hepatic phospholipid[23]	
Hepatic blood flow[24]	
Glomerular filtration rate[a,25]	
Vitamin and mineral stores[14]	

[a] In children only

This activity can be altered by many environmental factors, such as tobacco smoke[17] or chemicals.[18] Nutritional status can also influence rate of drug metabolism[14,19] and thus may modify drug response.

Water-soluble drugs and drug metabolites are chiefly distributed throughout body water and lean body mass. They are eliminated by the kidneys, and their rate of excretion is dependent on renal function, especially glomerular filtration rates. Tubular mechanisms are important for excretion of some drugs (e.g., penicillin).

Rate of drug elimination is often described by the elimination half-life ($t\frac{1}{2}$). However, half-life is also affected by volume of distribution. The term *plasma clearance* (Cl) better describes the rate of elimination, since it is independent of volume of distribution. It is usually expressed in units of milliliters per minute (ml/min).

PATHOPHYSIOLOGICAL CHANGES IN MALNUTRITION

The major pathophysiological changes that occur in severe protein/calorie malnutrition (PCM) that may effect drug kinetics are indicated in Table 4-1. It should be noted that changes in the gastrointestinal tract that affect drug absorption are not included, since absorption is discussed elsewhere in this book. It has been shown that body cell mass and fat are depleted[20,21] and that total body water increases, mainly because of an expansion of extracellular fluid volume.[21] These changes may increase the apparent volume of distribution of water-soluble drugs and diminish that of fat-soluble drugs. Plasma albumin concentrations fall in severe malnutrition, which may cause decreased binding of acidic drugs. There are, as yet, no data on the effect of poor diet on alpha-1 acid glycoprotein, which binds many basic drugs.

Certain hepatic changes have been described in malnutrition. Although fatty liver is commonly seen in children, it appears uncommon in adults.[14] Changes in routine liver function tests do not appear significant,[27] but these are blunt measurements of disordered function.

Other workers have demonstrated lower hepatic phospholipid content (mainly of the phosphatidyl ethanolamine fraction),[28] which may affect the integrity of membrane function necessary for efficient microsomal enzyme activity. In addition, lower cardiac output[24] may be accompanied by diminished hepatic blood flow, thus impairing elimination of drugs with higher intrinsic metabolic clearance.

While low glomerular filtration rate has been observed in children[25] this finding has not been confirmed in adults.[29] Therefore, it is likely that undernutrition is of little importance in renal elimination of drugs in the elderly, unless the aged kidney is more sensitive to nutritional deprivation.

Finally, many micronutrient deficiencies (including vitamins A, B, C, calcium, iron, and magnesium) that occur in undernutrition may retard hepatic drug metabolism since they form important components of enzymes and co-enzymes involved in such reactions.[19]

PHYSIOLOGICAL CHANGES WITH AGING

There are many physiological differences between young and elderly (Table 4-2) that should theoretically alter drug kinetics. Lean body mass and body water are lower in the elderly, both in absolute terms and as a proportion of total body weight. Water-soluble drugs should therefore distribute less widely and attain higher plasma concentrations in the elderly. Greater body fat stores may permit wider distribution of lipophilic drugs, which can prolong duration of action.

Serum albumin concentration is consistently lower in the aged, with important implications for binding of acidic drugs. It is not yet established whether α_1 acid glycoprotein concentration alters in senescence.

Although hepatic weight appears to decline with age, decline in function is not seen on routine biochemical liver function tests.[39] However, some,[39] but not all,[40] authors have reported higher bromosulphalein (BSP) retention in advanced age. Indocyanine green (ICG) retention is also higher.[41] The observation of lower liver blood flow in old age is compatible with higher BSP and ICG retention.[41] On this basis, elimination of certain drugs with high intrinsic clearance (e.g., propranolol) may be less rapid in older subjects.

It has been consistently observed that glomerular filtration rate and tubular function decline with age, suggesting lower renal drug elimination rate in the elderly.

These physiological changes form a solid basis for the premise that drug kinetics may be altered by aging. The most clear-cut and consistent changes of the above parameters are in renal function, suggesting that the most important age-related pharmacokinetic changes occur in renal drug elimination. This thesis has been borne out by evidence acquired so far, as will be discussed later.

Table 4-2. Age-Related Physiological Changes

Decrease	Increase
Total body water[30]	Body fat[30]
Lean body mass[31]	
Serum albumin[32]	
Splanchnic blood flow[33,42]	
Liver mass[34]	
Renal plasma flow[35]	
Glomerular filtration rate[36]	
Renal tubular function[37,38]	

PHARMACOKINETICS IN MALNUTRITION

Animal Studies

The effect of nutrition on drug kinetics has been widely studied in animals and has been mainly confined to examination of hepatic drug metabolizing enzyme systems in vitro. Particularly, attention has been devoted to the microsomal mixed-function oxidase pathway.[19] This work was prompted by clinical need to discern the effect of malnutrition on drug metabolism, but also by the possibility of nutrition having a role in carcinogenesis (by affecting the rate of metabolism of carcinogens or of production of carcinogenic metabolites). Reports concerning the effect of malnutrition on drug metabolism shall be briefly reviewed.

Macronutrient Deficiencies Lipid appears important in drug metabolism. It comprises a significant fraction of the smooth endoplasmic reticulum. Phospholipid is necessary for maintaining the structure of the microsomal membrane[43] and plays a specific role in the MFO system.[19]

Fat-free diet produces lower cytochrome P450 and drug-metabolizing enzyme activity compared with normal diet including essential free fatty acids.[45] Polyunsaturated fat may also be necessary in the diet to permit enzyme induction.[46] Also, choline deficiency lowers microsomal phospholipid content and hydrolase activity.[47]

Diets deficient in protein are known to reduce in vitro drug oxidation and also to increase in vivo drug half-lives.[48] These phenomena occur with poor-quality protein diet[49] and appear due to modification of hepatic MFO enzyme activity,[50] perhaps partly due to alteration of the action of phosphatidylcholine in the system.[19]

Carbohydrate-rich diet diminished biphenyl 4-hydroxylase and cytochrome P450 content in rat liver,[51] and in another study prolonged barbiturate sleep time in mice.[52] It is not understood how high-saccharide diet produces these effects.

Micronutrient Deficiencies An association has been observed between vitamin A deficiency and low cytochrome P450 enzyme activity in rats,[53] possibly due to an effect on membrane integrity.

Riboflavin is of special interest since it forms an integral part of flavoprotein reductase. Observations that riboflavin deficiency in animals can produce variable effects on substrate metabolism[54] have led to the hypothesis that certain pathways of microsomal metabolism may be flavin dependent (e.g., 3-4 benzopyrene hydroxylation), whereas others may not be.[55,56]

Zannoni et al.[57] have reported slower in vivo drug metabolism and lower enzyme activity in scorbutic animals. Also, ascorbic acid deficiency may impair enzyme induction by organochloride pesticides.[58]

Mineral Deficiencies

Deficiencies of certain minerals, such as calcium and iron, are relatively common in elderly humans,[13] and the effects of such deficiencies have been studied in animals. Calcium-deficient diets have been noted to produce oxidative rates for hexobarbital and p-nitrobenzoic acid less than half those in control animals.[59]

Table 4-3. Effect of Malnutrition on Drug Protein Binding

Decrease	No change
Chloramphenicol[64]	Streptomycin[72]
Digoxin[65]	Sulfafurazole[68]
Phenylbutazone[66]	
Salicylate[67]	
Sulfadiazine[22]	
Tetracycline[69]	
Thiopentone[70]	
Warfarin[71]	

Magnesium deficiency is also associated with impared microsomal enzyme activity.[60,61]

Microsomal enzyme activity appears to be greater in iron deficiency.[62] There is no firm explanation for this observation, although it has been suggested that iron deficiency may lessen NADPH-dependent degradation of endoplasmic membrane by NADP peroxidase enzymes.[63]

Clinical Studies

Most investigations of the effect of malnutrition on drug disposition have been conducted in children and young male adults suffering from protein/calorie malnutrition (PCM) in developing regions.[14] The effects of malnutrition on drug distribution and elimination are shown in Tables 4-3, 4-4, and 4-5 respectively. Unfortunately, these studies did not include any elderly persons, so there is no direct evidence of the effect of malnutrition on drug handling in this age group.

Macronutrient Deficiency The most notable alteration in drug kinetics in malnutrition is reduced protein binding (Table 4-3). Differences are usually large, in the order of 20% or more. In the case of highly bound drugs, reduced protein binding implies a significantly greater free-drug concentration in malnutrition. It would, therefore, be appropriate to compare free-drug kinetics in this context, but so far this comparison has not been performed.

Lower drug binding is due to lower serum albumin concentration. On the other hand, binding of streptomycin is unchanged, presumably because it also binds to globulins, which attain higher concentration in malnutrition.[14]

Volume of distribution is little altered by malnutrition (Table 4-4). This finding is surprising for water-soluble drugs such as phenazone, especially in groups of subjects with edema.[14] The distribution volume may not alter because the increase in extracellular water is matched by a decrease in intracellular water in malnutrition.[21]

Table 4-4. Effect of Malnutrition on Drug Volume of Distribution

No change	Decrease	Increase
Phenazone[73,75]	Tetracycline[69]	Phenylbutazone[66]
Streptomycin[72]		
Sulfadiazine[22]		
Sulfafurazole[68]		

Table 4-5. Effect of Malnutrition on Drug Half-Life and Clearance

	Decrease	Increase	No change
Half-life	Chloramphenicol[a,76]	Penicillin[a,77]	Phenazone[b,74]
	Phenazone[c,74]	Phenazone[73,75]	Sulfafurazole[68]
	Phenylbutazone[66]		Streptomycin[72]
	Sulfadiazine[22]		
	Tetracycline[69]		
Clearance	Phenazone[73,75]	Phenylbutazone[66]	Sulfafurazole[68]
		Sulfadiazine[22]	

[a] Exact half-life values not given
[b] In malnourished adults with edema
[c] In underweight adults

In the studies on half-life in malnutrition (Table 4-5), phenazone is the only drug included that undergoes oxidative metabolism. In children, phenazone half-life is prolonged,[73,75] whereas in adults it is similar or shorter.[74] The latter observation may be related to environmental factors, such as smoking and exposure to pesticides.[74] Shorter half-life of drugs excreted by the kidneys, such as tetracyclines and sulfadiazine, may reflect reduced protein binding rather than enhanced renal elimination per se. Less-rapid penicillin excretion in children is possible due to lower renal tubular elimination.

There is little data on the effect of malnutrition on drug clearance (Table 4-5). Phenazone clearance is lower, suggesting diminished microsomal oxidative capacity in malnutrition. The results for sulfadiazine and sulfafurazole (drugs that are partly acetylated but mainly excreted by the kidney) are apparently contradictory. However, these results are not strictly comparable because of differences in mode of administration, protein binding, urine pH, and also possibly acetylation phenotype distribution.

In summary, protein/calorie malnutrition is a complex, heterogenous deficiency state, and may have no simple effect on drug kinetics apart from that on albumin binding. The research to date is only preliminary. Further investigations are required, examining free-drug kinetics after intravenous administration and using more data points and longer sampling periods. Obviously, subject selection needs to be carefully performed, as indicated by Krishnaswamy and Naider.[74]

Micronutrient Deficiencies Little attention has been directed toward examination of drug metabolism in clinical micronutrient deficiency states. Although O'Malley and Stevenson[78] reported unchanged half-life, others[79] demonstrated higher phenazone clearance in iron deficiency. The degree of anemia and iron deficiency was so small in the latter study that the difference in phenazone clearance may have been for some other reason. However, good correlation was noted between transferrin saturation and phenazone clearance. O'Malley and Stevenson examined phenazone metabolism in patients before and after iron replacement therapy.[78] These subjects were more anemic (mean hemoglobin 52%). Half-life did not change with correction of anemia. Results of this better-designed study may be more meaningful.

Smithard and Langman[80] have also investigated the effect of vitamin supplementation on phenazone metabolism in elderly patients admitted to a geriatric

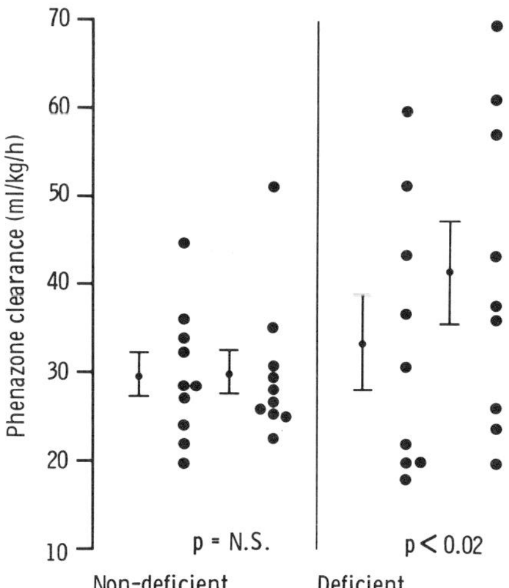

Fig. 4-1.   Effect of vitamin C treatment on phenazone clearance in subjects with normal and deficient vitamin C concentrations. Adapted with permission from Smithard DJ, Langman MJS: The effect of vitamin supplementation upon antipyrine metabolism in the elderly. Br J Clin Pharmacol 5:181–85, 1978.

ward. Drug clearance was measured along with leucocyte ascorbic acid and plasma vitamin A concentrations before and after two weeks of multivitamin supplementation. Results for clearance in those with normal and low vitamin C concentrations are shown in Figure 4-1. There was no difference between basal values in both groups. After vitamin treatment, clearance rose only in the scorbutic group, suggesting that correction of vitamin C deficiency enhances rate of metabolism. On the other hand, this interesting finding does not outrule an effect of general nutritional improvement in subjects in whom subnormal vitamin C concentrations may have been a marker of more general nutritional deficiency. Also, if repletion of vitamin C status was alone responsible for these changes in phenazone metabolism, one would expect that such changes (in comparison with the normal group) would be from a lower to a similar value (as reported in animals),[57] rather than from similar to higher values, as in this study. Some other factors, therefore, may have been responsible for the results observed.

AGING AND DRUG DISPOSITION

Elucidation of an effect of aging on drug metabolism in animals is difficult. It is expensive to keep animals into old age in standard conditions. Not surprisingly, investigation in this field has been limited.

Table 4-6. Effect of Aging on Protein Binding of Drugs

Decrease	No change	Increase
Diazepam[92]	Carbenoxolone[101]	Lidocaine[a,114]
Lorazepam[93]	Clobazam[102]	
Meperidine[94,95]	Chlordiazepoxide[103]	
Penicillin[96]	Chlormethiazole[104]	
Phenytoin[97]	Desmethyldiazepam[105]	
Theophylline[98]	Diazepam[106]	
Tolbutamide[99]	Flurazepam[107]	
Warfarin[100]	Maprotiline[108]	
	Phenobarbital[96]	
	Phenylbutazone[108]	
	Phenytoin[96]	
	Propranolol[110,111]	
	Quinidine[112]	
	Salicylate[109]	
	Sulfadiazine[109]	
	Warfarin[113]	

[a] Bound to α_1 acid glycoprotein

Investigations in Animals

Kato et al.[81] initially observed that meprobamate elimination half-life was longer in older rats. Results of further investigation similarly indicated that, in aged rats, rate of metabolism of pentobarbital, meprobamate, and carisoprodol was less rapid in vivo and in microsomal preparations.[82] The same investigators later demonstrated an age-related decline in both in vitro drug metabolism and microsomal enzyme activity.[83,84] Rate of in vivo drug elimination showed a parallel change with age.[85] Although these findings have been confirmed by some authors,[86] other reports have indicated no such change in drug metabolism in aged rats.[87,88] Studies in mice have similarly yielded conflicting results.[89,90]

There is no good explanation for the interstudy differences observed. However, they may be due to differences in feed and other environmental factors that can affect rate of drug metabolism.[91] Environmental and animal strain selection needs to be strictly standardized to permit valid comparison of such data.

Clinical Investigations

The effects of senescence on drug kinetics have by now been widely examined. It is pertinent to indicate that all of these studies are cross-sectional, comparing young and elderly adult groups. Thus, age is only one of many possible differences between such groups, such as dietary habits, smoking, and drug intake, that might affect drug kinetics.

Obviously, careful selection can obviate the potential effect of many of these factors. Despite their shortcomings, cross-sectional investigations have indicated some important kinetic differences between young and elderly, which shall now be discussed.

Protein Binding   Serum albumin concentrations are lower in the aged.[32]

Table 4-7. Effect of Aging on Volume of Distribution of Drugs

No change	Increase	Decrease
Acetaminophen[116]	Chlordiazepoxide[103,127]	Acetaminophen[135]
Ampicillin[117]	Chlormethiazole[128]	Acetanilide[136]
Amylobarbital[118]	Desmethyldiazepam[129]	Cimetidine[137]
Carbenozolone[101]	Diazepam[106]	Digoxin[138]
Clobazam[102]	Lidocaine[130]	Ethanol[139]
Desmethyldiazepam[105]	Nitrazepam[131]	Lorazepam[140]
Diazepam[119]	Oxazepam[132]	Meperidine[141]
Lidocaine[114]	Prazosin[133]	Phenazone[123,142,143]
Lorazepam[93]	Salicylate[134]	Propicillin[144]
Nitrazepam[120]	Tolbutamide[99]	Quinine[125]
Pancuronium[121]		Theophylline[98]
Phenazone[122]		
Phenylbutazone[116,123]		
Propranolol[124]		
Quinidine[112]		
Salicylate[125]		
Sulfamethizole[116]		
Theophylline[126]		

Protein binding of acidic drugs is closely related to serum albumin concentration,[97,100] and thus binding of many drugs is lower in old age (Table 4-6). In addition, multidrug therapy can cause displacement of such drugs as phenylbutazone, producing greater free-drug concentration.[109] However, the significance of lower drug binding in vitro or in single-dose studies in old age is not certain, since such differences do not necessarily imply higher free steady-state drug concentration.[115] Examination of age-related free-drug kinetics, especially after chronic dosing, would help clarify the importance of lower albumin binding.

Volume of Distribution The effect of old age on volume of distribution, shown in Table 4-7, is variable, with interstudy differences for certain drugs, such as acetaminophen and diazepam. However, in accordance with theoretical predictions, the general tendency is for fat-soluble drugs to have a higher, and water-soluble drugs a lower, volume of distribution in the elderly.

Volume of distribution is mainly a mathematical concept and says nothing of distribution to site of action. Altered regional distribution may be important in geriatric patients. Thus, greater sensitivity to such drugs as diazepam[145] and nitrazepam[120] may be due to greater blood/brain barrier permeability.

Drug Metabolism Tables 4-8 and 4-9 indicate that rate of drug metabolism as denoted by half-life or plasma clearance is generally either unchanged or lower in older subjects. However, no clear-cut pattern emerges. The effect of aging on microsomal enzyme metabolism of such drugs as phenazone, chlordiazepoxide, chlormethiazole, desmethyldiazepam, diazepam, and propranolol varies considerably. The same is true for drugs metabolized by nonmicrosomal systems, such as acetaminophen, carbenoxolone, isoniazid, and ethanol. Greater clearance of phenytoin and tolbutamide in old age may be an effect of lower protein binding[97,99] rather than altered metabolism per se.

This apparently complex effect of aging on human drug metabolism has some explanations. Some evidence suggests that environmental factors have a more

Table 4-8. Effect of Aging on Half-Life of Metabolized Drugs

Increase	No change
Acetanilide[146]	Acetaminophen[116]
Amylobarbital[118]	Acetanilide[136]
Carbenoxolone[101]	Chlordiazepoxide[127]
Clobazam[102]	Chlormethiazole[128]
Chlordiazepoxide[103]	Diazepam[119]
Desmethyldiazepam[105,129]	Imipramine[147]
Desmethylimiprimine[147]	Isoniazid[146]
Diazepam[106]	Lorazepam[93,140]
Indocyanine green[148]	Meperidine[141]
Lidocaine[114,130]	Metoprolol[150]
Nitrazepam[131]	Morphine[151]
Nortriptyline[149]	Nitrazepam[120]
Phenazone[122,143,152]	Oxazepam[132]
Prazosin[133]	Phenazone[143,148]
Propranolol[124]	Phenylbutazone[116,152]
Salicylate[134]	Propranolol[42]
	Temazepam[153]
	Theophylline[98,126]
	Warfarin[113]

powerful influence on drug metabolism, which may distort or override any effect of aging. For instance, Vestal et al.[142] demonstrated that only a small proportion (3%) of the decline in phenazone clearance in the elderly was due to aging, a greater effect being due to smoking (12%), with the remainder unexplained. These investigators later demonstrated that phenazone[148] and propranolol[42] clearance fell with age in smokers, but not in nonsmokers. Smoking was associated with a higher rate of metabolism in young people alone. They concluded that smoking accelerated drug metabolism by enzyme induction; this effect was manifest in the young, but not in the aged. These and other data[111,125] suggest that drug-metabolizing enzyme induction is blunted in old age, although other evidence contradicts this theory.[126] Also, subject selection is important; it has been demonstrated that the rate of phenazone metabolism in the elderly is more rapid in hospitalized patients than in healthy subjects.[143] This finding is important, since age-related kinetic studies often compare drug metabolism in healthy young and hospitalized elderly subjects. Differences observed may, therefore, be due to disease or hospitalization rather than to aging per se. The evidence to date thus points to a hypothesis that many putative age-related differences in drug metabolism may reflect altered environment or different response to environment rather than the aging process. Subjects must be rigorously selected to minimize these environmental distortions.

Although therefore of doubtful gerontological significance, altered drug metabolism in more casually selected elderly patients is of clinical importance if such results can be extrapolated to the general clinical situation. Thus, greater toxicity of some metabolized drugs, such as chlordiazepoxide,[157] in elderly patients may be due to a lower rate of metabolism in these patients, compared with the rate of metabolism in younger subjects in whom the standard drug dosage was calculated.

Renal Drug Excretion Renal drug elimination is consistently lower in elderly groups in all the studies shown in Table 4-10. These findings are consistent

Table 4-9. Effect of Aging on Clearance of Metabolized Drugs

Decrease	No change	Increase
Acetaminophen[135]	Acetaminophen[116]	Phenytoin[97]
Carbenoxolone[101]	Acetanilide[136]	Tobutamide[99]
Clobazam[a,102]	Diazepam[106,119]	
Chlordiazepoxide[103,127]	Diclofenac[154]	
Chlormethiazole[128]	Ethanol[139]	
Desmethyldiazepam[a,129]	Lidocaine[114,130]	
Desmethyldiazepam[105]	Lorazepam[93,140]	
Diazepam[92]	Nitrazepam[131]	
Indocyanine green[148]	Oxazepam[132]	
Norepinephrine[155]	Phenazone[b,143]	
Nortriptyline[149]	Phenazone[148]	
Phenazone[142,143,152]	Prazosin[133]	
Propranolol[124]	Propranolol[42,110]	
Phenylbutazone[123,152]	Salicylate[125,134]	
Quinidine[156]	Theophylline[126]	
Quinine[125]	Warfarin[113]	

[a] In males only; no change in females
[b] In elderly hospitalized patients

with predictions based on physiological data in Table 4-2 showing a decline in renal function with age. Elimination of drugs that are mainly dependent on glomerular filtration is lower in the elderly. Digoxin, quinidine, and sulphamethizole are good examples of this group. Rate of excretion of such drugs as penicillin, ampicillin, and procainamide, which is partly dependent on tubular function, is also lower in old age.

This phenomenon of lower average renal drug elimination is of undoubted clinical importance and implies that maintenance doses of these drugs ought to be reduced in the aged, including those with normal blood urea and serum creatinine. An important point is that the range of drug clearance values in such subjects is wide, so that some individuals may require under half, and others the full, adult dose.[138] Individualization of dosage is therefore necessary, especially for drugs with low therapeutic ratio, such as lithium or gentamicin.

SUMMARY AND CONCLUSION

The importance of the effect of malnutrition in humans is not yet established. Furthermore, disparity between findings in animals (which generally show diminished metabolism) and those in humans (which show no consistent pattern) have many explanations. For example, studies in animals have mainly been conducted in vitro,[19] while those in humans have been performed in vivo. Diminished MFO activity in vitro need not imply lower systemic drug clearance, since such diminished activity need not be the rate-limiting step in drug elimination. In this respect, examination of rate of metabolism in vivo in animals would permit more meaningful comparison with human data.

Evidence regarding the effect of malnutrition on drug disposition in humans is, as yet, preliminary, and, indeed, much of this evidence may be somewhat

Table 4-10. Effect of Aging on Renal Drug Elimination[a]

Decrease	Decrease
Acetylprocainamide[158]	Lithium[165,166]
Ampicillin[117]	Pancuronium[167]
Atenolol[110]	Penicillin[168,169]
Cefuroxime[167]	Phenobarbital[170]
Cephradine[159]	Practolol[171]
Cephazolin[159]	Procainamide[158]
Cimetidine[137]	Propicillin[144]
Digoxin[138,160]	Quinidine[112]
Dihydrostreptomycin[161]	Sulphamethizole[116]
Doxycycline[162]	Tetracycline[161,172]
Gentamicin[163]	
Kanamycin[164]	

[a] As indicated by elimination half-life and/or clearance

misleading because of possible effects of disparate factors, such as concomitant disease states, edema, and altered protein binding in many of the studies concerned. Factors such as these must be considered before one can make definitive statements regarding the effect of malnutrition on drug disposition in humans and compare such effect with animal data.

Widespread investigation of drug kinetics in old age has yielded some evidence of definite trends, such as lower binding of drugs to albumin and impaired renal drug clearance. For reasons previously discussed, the latter change is of particular clinical importance. The effect of aging on hepatic metabolism, however, is variable and influenced by environmental factors.

There are some indications that malnutrition may be one such important modifying factor, but this possibility has never been adequately investigated. There are reasons why little attention has been devoted to the possible interaction of nutrition and aging on drug metabolism. Elderly people are least common in regions where malnutrition is endemic. Conflicting evidence regarding the effect of poor diet on drug metabolism in young people has not excited extension of such work to include the elderly. Although dietary deficiency is relatively common in the aged in developed countries,[173-175] frank malnutrition is less common,[176] possibly because of reduced dietary demands.[13] Thus, in Western society, there is little opportunity and no urgent clinical need to assess the effect of malnutrition on drug disposition in senescence. However, poor nutrition and altered dietary habit may indeed contribute to some of the complex changes seen in drug metabolism in old age. This possibility deserves further investigation to help increase our knowledge of the relationship of aging to drug metabolism.

REFERENCES

1. Lamy PP, Kitler ME: Drugs and the geriatric patient. J Am Geriat Assoc 19:23–33, 1971.
2. Dans PE, Kerr, MR: Gerontology and geriatrics in medical education. New Engl J Med 300: 228–232, 1979.

3. Wilson LA, Lawson IR, Braws W: Multiple disorders in the elderly: A clinical and statistical study. Lancet 2:841–843, 1962.
4. Rowe JW: Clinical research on aging: Strategies and directions. New Engl J Med 297:1332–1336, 1977.
5. Hurwitz N: Predisposing factors in adverse reactions to drugs. Br Med J 1:536–539, 1969.
6. Seidl LG, Thornton GF, Smith JW, Cluff LE: Studies on the epidemiology of adverse drug reactions. 3. Reactions in patients in a general medical service. Bull Johns Hopkins Hosp 119:299–315, 1966.
7. Klein LE, German PS, Levine DM: Adverse drug reactions among the elderly: A reassessment. J. Am Ger Soc 29:525–530, 1981.
8. Crooks J, O'Malley K, Stevenson IH: Pharmacokinetics in the elderly. Clin Pharmacokin 1:280–296, 1976.
9. O'Malley K, Laher M, Cusack B, Kelly JG: Clinical pharmacology and the elderly patient. In Denham, MJ (ed): The Treatment of Medical Problems in the Elderly. Lancaster, England, MTP Press, 1980.
10. Richey DP, Bender AD: Pharmacokinetic consequences of aging. Am Rev Pharmacol Toxicol 17:49–65, 1977.
11. Triggs EJ, Nation RL: Pharmacokinetics in the aged: A review. J Pharmacokin Biopharm 2:387–418, 1975.
12. Vestal RE: Drug use in the elderly: A review of problems and special considerations. Drugs 16:358–382, 1978.
13. Munro HN: Nutrition and aging. Br Med Bull 37:83–88, 1981.
14. Krishnaswamy K: Drug metabolism and pharmacokinetics in malnutrition. Clin Pharmacokin 3:216–240, 1978.
15. Boobis AR, Davies DS: Pharmacokinetics. Hosp Update 7:453–460, 1981.
16. Greenblatt DJ, Koch-Weser J: Clinical pharmacokinetics. New Engl J Med 293:702–705, 964–969, 1975.
17. Jusko WJ: Role of tobacco smoking in pharmacokinetics. J. Pharmacokin Biopharm 6:7–39, 1978.
18. Alvares AP: Interaction between environmental chemicals and drug biotransformation in man. Clin Pharmacokin 3:462–477, 1978.
19. Campbell TC, Hayes JR: Role of nutrition in the drug-metabolizing enzyme system. Pharmacol Rev 26:171–197, 1974.
20. Alleyne GAO: Mineral metabolism in protein calorie malnutrition. In Olson RE (ed): Protein Calorie Malnutrition. New York, Academic Press, 1975.
21. Shizgal HM: The effect of malnutrition on body composition. Surg Gynecol Obstet 152:22–26, 1981.
22. Shastri RA, Krishnaswamy K: Metabolism of sulphadiazine in malnutrition. Br J Clin Pharmacol 7:69–73, 1979.
23. Chaplin MD, Mannering GJ: Role of phospholipids in the hepatic microsomal drug-metabolizing system. Mol Pharmacol 6:631–640, 1970.
24. Alleyne GAO: Cardiac function in severely malnourished Jamaican children. Clin Sci 30:553–562, 1966.
25. Alleyne GAO: The effect of severe PCM on the renal function of Jamaican children. Paediatrics 39:400–411, 1967.
26. Gapolan C, Krishnaswamy K: Famine oedema. Prog Food Nut Sci 1:207–224, 1975.
27. Kinnear AA, Pretorins PJ: Liver function in kwashiorkor. Br Med J 1:1528–1530, 1956.
28. Chatterjee KK, Mukherjee KL: Phospholipids of the liver in children suffering from protein-calorie undernutrition. Br J Nutr 22:145–151, 1968.

29. Srikantia SG, Gopalan C: Renal function in nutritional oedema. Ind J Med Res 47:467–470, 1959.
30. Edelman IS, Leibman J: Anatomy of body water and electrolytes. Am J Med 27:256–277, 1959.
31. Forbes GB, Reina JC: Adult lean body mass declines with age: Some longitudinal observations. Metabolism 19:653–663, 1970.
32. Greenblatt DJ: Reduced serum albumin concentration in the elderly: A report from the Boston collaborative drug surveillance program. J Am Geriat Soc 27:20–22, 1979.
33. Sherlock S, Bearn AG, Billing BH, Paterson JCS: Splanchnic blood flow in man by the bromosulphalein method: The relation of peripheral plasma bromosulphalein level to the calculated flow. J Lab Clin Med 35:923–932, 1950.
34. Calloway NO, Foley CF, Lagerbloom P: Uncertainties in geriatric data. 2. Organ size. J Am Geriat Soc 13:20–26, 1965.
35. Davies DF, Shock NW: Age changes in glomerular filtration rate, effective renal plasma flow and tubular excretory capacity in adult males. J Clin Invest 29:496–507, 1950.
36. Rowe JW, Andres R, Tobin JD, et al.: The effect of age on creatinine clearance in man: a cross-sectional and longitudinal study. J Gerontol 31:155–163, 176.
37. Miller JH, McDonald RK, Shock NW: Age changes in the maximal rate of renal tubular reabsorption of glucose. J Gerontol 7:196–200, 1952.
38. Rowe JW, Shock NW, De Fronzo RA: The influence of age on renal response to water deprivation in man. Nephron 17:270–278, 1976.
39. Thompson EN, Williams R: Effect of age on liver function with particular rerference to bromosulphalein excretion. Gut 6:266–269, 1965.
40. Koff RS, Garvey AJ, Burney SW, Bell B: Absence of age effect on sulphobromophthalein retention in healthy man. Gastroenterology 65:300–302, 1973.
41. Kitani K: Functional aspects of the aging liver. In Platt D. (ed): Liver and Ageing, Stuttgart/New York, Schattauer Verlag, 1977, pp 5–19.
42. Vestal RE, Wood AJJ, Branch RA, et al.: Effects of age and cigarette smoking on propranolol disposition. Clin Pharmacol Ther 26:8–15, 1979.
43. Glaumann H, Dallner G: Lipid composition and turnover of rough and smooth microsomal membranes in rat liver. J Lipid Res 9:720–729, 1968.
44. Vore M, Hamilton JG, Lu Hyh: Organic solvent extraction of liver microsomal lipid. 1. The requirements of lipid for 3,4-benzopyrene hydroxylase. Biochem Biophys Res Comm 56:1038–1044, 1974.
45. Norred WP, Wade AE: Dietary fatty acid–induced alteration of hepatic microsomal drug metabolism. Biochem Pharmacol 21:2887–2897, 1972.
46. Marshall WJ, McLean AEM: A requirement for dietary lipids for induction of cytochrome P-450 by phenobarbitone in rat liver microsomal fraction. Biochem J 122:569–573, 1971.
47. Cooper SD, Feuer G: Effects of drugs or hepatotoxins on the relation between drug metabolizing activity and phospholipids in hepatic microsomes during choline deficiency. Toxicol Appl Pharmacol 25:7–19, 1973.
48. Kato R, Oshima T, Tomizawa S: Toxicity and metabolism of drugs in relation to dietary protein. Jap J Pharmacol 18:356–366, 1968.
49. Miranda CL, Webb RE: Effects of dietary protein quality on drug metabolism in the rat. J Nut 103:1425–1430, 1973.
50. Hayes JR, Campbell TC: Effect of protein deficiency on the inducibility of the hepatic microsomal drug-metabolizing enzyme system. 3. Effect of 3-methyl-cholanthrene induction on activity and binding kinetics. Biochem Pharmacol 23:1721–1731, 1974.

51. Dickerson JWT, Basu TK, Parke DV: Activity of drug metabolizing enzymes in the liver of growing rats fed on diets high in sucrose, glucose, fructose or an equimolar mixture of glucose and fructose. Proc Nutr Soc 30:27A–28A, 1971.
52. Strother A, Throckmorton JK, Herzer C: The influence of high sugar consumption by mice on the duration of action of barbiturates and in vitro metabolism of barbiturates aniline and p-nitroanisole. J Pharmacol Exp Ther 179:490–498, 1971.
53. Becking GC: Vitamin A status and hepatic drug metabolism in the rat. Can J Physiol Pharmacol 56:6–11, 1973.
54. Catz CS, Juckau MR, Yaffe SJ: Effects of iron, riboflavin and iodide deficiencies on hepatic drug-metabolizing enzyme systems. J Pharmacol Exp Ther 174:197–205, 1970.
55. Shargel L, Mazel P: The effect of flavin on purified microsomal azoreductase. Toxicol Appl Pharmacol 12:317, 1968.
56. Shargel L, Mazel P: Effect of riboflavin deficiency on phenobarbital and 3-methylcholanthrene induction of microsomal drug-metabolizing enzymes of the rat. Biochem Pharmacol 22:2365–2373, 1973.
57. Zannoni VG, Flynn EJ, Lynch M: Ascorbic acid and drug metabolism. Biochem Pharmacol 21:1377–1392, 1972.
58. Wagstaff DJ, Street JC: Ascorbic acid deficiency and induction of hepatic microsomal hydroxylative enzymes by organochlorine pesticides. Toxicol Appl Pharmacol 19:10–19, 1971.
59. Dignell JV, Joiner PD, Hurwitz L: Impairment of hepatic drug metabolism in calcium deficiency. Biochem Pharmacol 15:971–976, 1966.
60. Becking GC, Morrison AB: Role of dietary magnesium in the metabolism of drugs by the NADPH-dependent rat liver microsomal enzymes. Biochem Pharmacol 19:2639–2644, 1970.
61. Peters MA, Fouts JR: The influence of magnesium and some other divalent cations on hepatic microsomal drug metabolism in vitro. Biochem Pharmacol 19:533–544, 1970.
62. Becking GC: Influence of dietary iron levels on hepatic drug metabolism in vivo and in vitro in the rat. Biochem Pharmacol 21:1585–1593, 1972.
63. Wills ED: Effects of iron overload on lipid peroxide formation and oxidative demethylation by the liver endoplasmic reticulum. Biochem Pharmacol 21:239–247, 1972.
64. Buchanan N, Van der Walt LA: Chloramphenicol binding to normal and kwashiorkor sera. Am J Clin Nutr 30:847–859, 1977.
65. Buchanan N, Van der Walt LA: The binding of digoxin to normal and kwashiorkor serum. J. Pharm Sci 65:914–916, 1976.
66. Krishnaswamy K, Ushasri V, Naidu AN: The effect of malnutrition on the pharmacokinetics of phenylbutazone. Clin Pharmacokin 6:152–159, 1981.
67. Eyberg C, Moodby GP, Buchanan N: Salicylate binding studies using normal serum/plasma and kwashiorkor serum. S Afr Med J 48:2564–2567, 1974.
68. Shastri RA: Kinetics of sulphafurazole in undernutrition. Br J Clin Pharmacol 10:499–502, 1980.
69. Shastri RA, Krishnaswamy K: Undernutrition and tetracycline half-life. Clin Chim Acta 66:157–164, 1976.
70. Buchanan N, Van der Walt LA: Thiopentone binding to normal and kwashiorkor sera. Br J Anaes 49:247–250, 1977.
71. Buchanan N, Van der Walt LA: Warfarin binding in kwashiorkor. Hlth J 94:128, 1977.
72. Prasad JS, Krishnaswamy K: Streptomycin pharmacokinetics in malnutrition. Chemotherapy 24:333–337, 1978.

73. Homeida M, Karrar ZA, Roberts CJC: Drug metabolism in malnourished children: A study with antipyrine. Arch Dis Child 54:299–302, 1979.
74. Krishnaswamy K, Naidu N: Microsomal enzymes in malnutrition as determined by plasma half-life of antipyrine. Br Med J 1:538–540, 1977.
75. Narang RK, Mehta S, Mathur VS: Pharmacokinetic study of antipyrine in malnourished children. Am J Clin Nutr 30:1979–1982, 1977.
76. Mehta S, Kalsi HK, Jayaraman S, Mathur VS: Chloramphenicol metabolism in children with protein-calorie malnutrition. Am J Clin Nutr 28:977–981, 1975.
77. Bolme P, Gebre Ab T, Hadgu P, et al.: Absorption and elimination of penicillin in children with malnutrition. Ethiop Med J 18:151–157, 1980.
78. O'Malley K, Stevenson IH: Iron deficiency anaemia and drug metabolism. J. Pharm Pharmacol 25:338–340, 1973.
79. Langman MJS, Smithard DJ: Antipyrine metabolism in iron deficiency. Br J Clin Pharmacol 4:631P, 1977.
80. Smithard DJ, Langman MJS: The effect of vitamin supplementation upon antipyrine metabolism in the elderly. Br J Clin Pharmacol 5:181–185, 1978.
81. Kato R, Chiesara E, Frontino G: Induced increase of meprobamate metabolism in rats pretreated with phenobarbital or phenaglycodol in relation to age. Experientia 17:520–521, 1961.
82. Kato R, Vassanelli P, Frontino G, Chiesara E: Variation in the activity of liver microsomal drug-metabolizing enzymes in rats in relation to the age. Biochem Pharmacol 13:1037–1051, 1964.
83. Kato R, Takanaka A: Effect of phenobarbital on electron transport system, oxidation and reduction of drugs in liver microsomes of rats of different age. J Biochem 63:406–408, 1968.
84. Kato R, Takanaka A: Metabolism of drugs in old rats. 1. Activities of NADPH-linked electron transport and drug-metabolizing enzyme systems in liver microsomes of old rats. Jap J Pharmacol 18:381–388, 1968.
85. Kato R, Takanaka A: Metabolism of drugs in old rats. 2. Metabolism in vivo and effect of drugs in old rats. Jap J. Pharmacol 18:389–396, 1968.
86. Baird MB, Nicolosi RJ, Massie HR, Samis HV: Microsomal mixed-function oxidase activity and senescence. 1. Hexobarbital sleep time and induction of components of the microsomal enzyme system in rats of different ages. Exp Gerontol 10:89–99, 1975.
87. Birnbaum LS, Baird, MB: Induction of hepatic mixed function oxidases in senescent rodents. Exp Gerontol 13:299–303, 1978.
88. Adelman RC: Age-dependent effects in enzyme induction: A biochemical expression of aging. Exp Gerontol 6:75–87, 1971.
89. Kato R, Takanaka A, Onoda KT: Studies on age difference in mice for the activity of drug-metabolizing enzymes of liver microsomes. Jap J Pharmacol 20:572–576, 1970.
90. Birnbaum LS: Altered hepatic drug metabolism in senescent mice. Exp Gerontol 15:-259–267, 1980.
91. Vessel ES, Maxhang C, White WJ, et al.: Environmental and genetic factors affecting the response of laboratory animals to drugs. Fed Proc 35:1125–1132, 1976.
92. Macklon AF, James O, Rawlins MD: Hepatic metabolism of diazepam in relation to age. Clin Sci 56:12p, 1979.
93. Kraus JW, Desmond PV, Marshall JP, et al.: Effects of aging and liver disease on disposition of lorazepam. Clin Pharmacol Ther 24:411–419, 1978.
94. Mitchard M: Drug distribution in the elderly. In Crooks J, Stevenson IH (eds): Drugs and the Elderly. London, Macmillan, 1979.

95. Mather LE, Tucker GT, Pflug AE, et al.: Meperidine kinetics in man; Intravenous injection in surgical patients and volunteers. Clin Pharmacol Ther 17:21–30, 1975.
96. Bender AD, Post A, Meier JP, et al.: Plasma protein binding of drugs as a function of age in adult human subjects. J Pharm Sci 64:1711–1713, 1975.
97. Hayes MJ, Langman MJS, Short AH: Changes in drug metabolism with increasing age. 2. Phenytoin clearance and protein binding. Br J Clin Pharmacol 2:73–79, 1975.
98. Antal EJ, Kramer PA, Mercik SA, et al.: Theophylline pharmacokinetics in advanced age. Br J Clin Pharmacol 12:637–645, 1981.
99. Miller AK, Adir J, Vestal RE: Effect of age on the pharmacokinetics of tolbutamide in man. Pharmacologist 19:128, 1977.
100. Hayes MJ, Langman MJS, Short AH: Changes in drug metabolism with increasing age. 1. Warfarin binding and plasma proteins. Br J Clin Pharmacol 2:69–72, 1975.
101. Hayes MJ, Sprackling M, Langman MJS: Changes in plasma clearance and protein binding of carbenoxolone with age, and their possible relationship with adverse drug effects. Gut 18:1054–1058, 1977.
102. Greenblatt DJ, Divoll M, Puri SK, et al.: Clobazam kinetics in the elderly. Br J Clin Pharmacol 12:631–636, 1981.
103. Roberts RK, Wilkinson GR, Branch RA, Sheuker S: Effect of age and parenchymal liver disease on the disposition and elimination of chlordiazepoxide (Librium). Gastroenterology 75:479–485, 1978.
104. Nation RL, Vine J, Triggs EJ, Learoyd B: Plasma levels of chlormethiazole and two metabolites after oral administration to young and aged human subjects. Eur J Clin Pharmacol 12:137–145, 1977.
105. Klotz U, Muller-Seydlitz P: Altered elimination of desmethyldiazepam in the elderly. Br J Clin Pharmacol 7:119–120, 1979.
106. Klotz U, Avant GR, Hoyampa A, et al.: The effects of age and liver disease on the disposition and elimination of diazepam in adult man. J Clin Invest 55:347–359, 1975.
107. Greenblatt DJ, Divoll M, Harmatz JS, et al.: Kinetics and clinical effects of flurazepam in young and elderly insomniacs. Clin Pharmacol Ther 30:475–486, 1981.
108. Braithwaite RA, Heard R, Snape A: Plasma protein binding of maprotiline in geriatric patients: Influence of acid flycoprotein. Br J Clin Pharmacol 6:448p–449p, 1978.
109. Wallace S, Whiting B, Runcie J: Factors affecting drug binding in plasma of elderly patients. Br J Clin Pharmacol 3:327–330, 1976.
110. Barber HE, Hawksworth GM, Petrie JC, et al.: Pharmacokinetics of atenolol and propranolol in young and elderly subjects. Br J Clin Pharmacol 12:118p–119p, 1981.
111. Feely J, Crooks J, Stevenson IH: The influence of age, smoking and hyperthyroidism on plasma propranolol steady-state concentration. Br J Clin Pharmacol 12:73–78, 1981.
112. Ochs HR, Greenblatt DJ, Woo E, Smith TW: Reduced quinidine clearance in elderly subjects. Am J Cardiol 42:481–485, 1978.
113. Shepherd AMM, Hewick DS, Moreland TA, Stevenson IH: Age as a determinant of sensitivity to warfarin. Br J Clin Pharmacol 4:315–320, 1977.
114. Cusack B, Kelly JG, Lavan J, et al.: Pharmacokinetics of lignocaine in the elderly. Br J Clin Pharmacol 9:293p–294p, 1980.
115. Klotz U: Pathophysiological and disease-induced changes in drug distribution volume. Pharmacokinetic implications. Clin Pharmacokin 1:204–218, 1976.
116. Triggs EJ, Nation RL, Long A, Ashley JJ: Pharmacokinetics in the elderly. Eur J Clin Pharmacol 8:55–62, 1975.
117. Triggs EJ, Johnson JM, Learoyd B: Absorption and disposition of ampicillin in the elderly. Eur J Clin Pharmacol 18:195–198, 1980.

118. Ritschel WA: Age-dependent disposition of amylobarbital: Analog computer evaluation. J Am Geriat Soc 26:540–543, 1978.
119. MacLeod SM, Giles HG, Bengert B, et al.: Age and gender-related differences in diazepam pharmacokinetics. J Clin Pharmacol 19:15–19, 1979.
120. Castledon CM, George CF, Marcer D, Hallett C: Increased sensitivity to nitrazepam in old age. Br Med J 1:10–12, 1977.
121. McLeod K, Hull CJ, Watson MJ: Effects of ageing on the pharmacokinetics of pancuronium. Br J Anaesth 51:435–438, 1979.
122. Liddell DE, Williams FM, Briant RH: Phenazone (antipyrine) metabolism and distribution in young and elderly adults. Clin Exp Pharmacol Physiol 2:481–487, 1975.
123. O'Malley K: Ph.D. thesis. University of Dundee, 1973.
124. Castleden CM, George CF: The effect of ageing on the hepatic clearance of propranolol. Br J Clin Pharmacol 7:49–54, 1979.
125. Salem SAM, Stevenson IH: Absorption kinetics of aspirin and quinine in elderly subjects. Br J Clin Pharmacol 4:397p, 1977.
126. Cusack B, Kelly JG, Lavan J, et al.: Theophylline kinetics in relation to age: The importance of smoking. Br J Clin Pharmacol 10:109–114, 1980.
127. Shader RI, Greenblatt DJ, Harmatz JS, et al.: Absorption and disposition of chlordiazepoxide in young and elderly male volunteers. J Clin Pharmacol 17:709–715, 1977.
128. Nation RL, Learoyd B, Barker J, Triggs EJ: The pharmacokinetics of chlormethiazole following intravenous administration in the aged. Eur J Clin Pharmacol 10:407–415, 1976.
129. Allen MD, Greenblatt DJ, Harmatz JS, Shader RI: Desmethyldiazepam kinetics in the elderly after oral prazepam. Clin Pharmacol Ther 28:196–202, 1980.
130. Nation RL, Triggs EJ, Selig M: Lignocaine kinetics in cardiac patients and aged subjects. Br J Clin Pharmacol 4:439–448, 1977.
131. Kangas L, Iisalo E, Kanto J, et al.: Human pharmacokinetics of nitrazepam: Effect of age and diseases. Eur J Clin Pharmacol 15:163–170, 1979.
132. Shull HJ, Wilkinson GR, Johnson R, Schenker S: Normal disposition of oxazepam in acute viral hepatitis and cirrhosis. Ann Int Med 84:420–425, 1976.
133. Rubin PC, Scott PJW, Reid JL: Prazosin disposition in young and elderly subjects. Br J Clin Pharmacol 12:401–404, 1981.
134. Cuny G, Royer RJ, Mur JM, et al.: Pharmacokinetics of salicylates in the elderly. Gerontology 25:49–55, 1979.
135. Fulton B, James O, Rawlins MD: The influence of age on the pharmacokinetics of paracetamol. Br J Clin Pharmacol 7:418p, 1979.
136. Playfer JR, Baty JD, Lamb J, et al.: Age-related differences in the disposition of acetanilide. Br J Clin Pharmacol 6:529–535, 1978.
137. Redolfi A, Borgogelli E, Lodola E: Blood level of cimetidine in relation to age. Eur J Clin Pharmacol 15:257–261, 1979.
138. Cusack B, Kelly JG, O'Malley K, et al.: Digoxin in the elderly: Pharmacokinetic consequences of old age. Clin Pharmacol Ther 25:772–776, 1979.
139. Vestal RE, McGuire EA, Tobin JD, et al.: Aging and ethanol metabolism. Clin Pharmacol Ther 21:343–354, 1977.
140. Greenblatt DJ, Allen MD, Locniskar A, et al.: Lorazepam kinetics in the elderly. Clin Pharmacol Ther 25:103–113, 1979.
141. Chan K, Mitchard M: Elevated plasma pethidine levels in elderly patients after intravenous administration. Proc Br Pharmacol Soc Meet C33, February 1978.
142. Vestal RE, Norris AH, Jordan D, et al.: Antipyrine metabolism in man: Influence of

age, alcohol, caffeine and smoking. Clin Pharmacol Ther 18:425–432, 1975.

143. Swift CG, Homeida M, Halliwell M, Roberts CJC: Antipyrine disposition and liver size in the elderly. Eur J Clin Pharmacol 14:149–152, 1978.

144. Simon C, Malerezyk V, Muller U, Muller G: Zur Pharmakokinetik von Propicillin bei geriatrischen Patienten im Vergleich zur jüngeren Erwachsenen. Deutsche Med Wochenschr 97:1999–2003, 1972.

145. Reidenberg MM, Levy M, Warner H, et al.: Relationship between diazepam dose, plasma level, age and central nervous system depression. Clin Pharmacol Ther 23:371–376, 1978.

146. Farah F, Taylor W, Rawlins MD, James O: Hepatic drug acetylation and oxidation: Effects of aging in man. Br Med J 2:155–156, 1977.

147. Nies A, Robinson DS, Friedman MJ, et al.: Relationship between age and tricyclic antidepressant plasma levels. Am J Psychiat 134:790–793, 1977.

148. Wood AJJ, Vestal RE, Wilkinson GR, et al.: Effect of aging and cigarette smoking on antipyrine and indocyanine green elimination. Clin Pharmacol Ther 26:16–20, 1979.

149. Dawling S, Crome P, Braithwaite RA, Lewis RR: Nortriptyline therapy in elderly patients: Dosage prediction after single-dose pharmacokinetic study. Eur J Clin Pharmacol 18:147–150, 1980.

150. Quarterman CP, Kendall MJ, Jack DB: The effect of age on the pharmacokinetics of metoprolol and its metabolites. Br J Clin Pharmacol 11:287–294, 1981.

151. Berkowitz BA, Ngai SH, Yong JC, et al.: The disposition of morphine in surgical patients. Clin Pharmacol Ther 17:629–635, 1975.

152. O'Malley K, Crooks J, Duke E, Stevenson IH: Effect of age and sex on human drug metabolism. Br Med J 3:607–609, 1971.

153. Briggs RS, Castleden CM, Kraft CA: Improved hypnotic treatment using chlormethiazole and temazepam. Br Med J 280:601–604, 1980.

154. Willis JV, Kendall MJ: Pharmacokinetic studies on diclofenac sodium in young and old volunteers. Scand J Rheumatol, suppl 22, pp 36–41, 1978.

155. Ester M, Skews H, Leonard P, et al.: Age-dependence of nor-adrenaline kinetics in normal subjects. Clin Sci 60:217–219, 1981.

156. Drayer DE, Hughes M, Lorenzo B, Reidenberg MM: Prevalence of high (3S)-3-hydroxyquinidine/quinidine ratios in serum, and clearance of quinidine in cardiac patients with age. Clin Pharmacol Ther 27:72–75, 1980.

157. Boston Collaborative Drug Surveillance Program: Clinical depression of the central nervous system due to diazepam and chlordiazepoxide in relation to cigarette smoking and age. New Engl J Med 288:277–280, 1973.

158. Reidenberg MM, Comacko M, Kluger J, Drayer DE: Aging and renal clearance of procainamide and acetylprocainamide. Clin Pharmacol Ther 28:732–735, 1980.

159. Simon C, Malerczyk V, Tenshert B, Mohlenbeck F: Die geriatrische Pharmacologie von Cefazolin, Cefradin und Sulfisomidin. Arzneim Forsch 26:1377–1382, 1976.

160. Ewy GA, Kapadia GC, Yao L, et al.: Digoxin metabolism in the elderly. Circulation 39:449–453, 1969.

161. Vartia KO, Leikola E: Serum levels of antibiotics in young and old subjects following administration of dihydrostreptomycin and tetracycline. J Gerontol 15:392–394, 1960.

162. Simon C, Malerczyk V, Englake H, et al.: Die Pharmakokinetik von Doxycylin bei Niereninsuffizienz und geriatrischen Patienten in Vergleich zur jüngeren Erwachsenen. Schweiz Med Wochenschr 105:1615–1620, 1975.

163. Lumholtz B, Kampmann J, Siersback-Nielsen K, Mølholm Hansen J: Dose regimen of kanamycin and gentamycin. Acta Med Scand 190:521–524, 1974.

164. Kristensen M, Mølholm Hansen J, Kampmann J, et al.: Drug elimination and renal function. J Clin Pharmacol 14:307–308, 1974.
165. Hewisk DS, Newbury P, Hopwood S, et al.: Age as a factor affecting lithium therapy. Br J Clin Pharmacol 4:201–205, 1977.
166. Lehmann K, Merton K: Die Elimination von Lithium in Abhängigkeit vom Lebensalter bei Gesunden und Niereninsuffizienten. Int J Clin Pharmacol 10:292–298, 1974.
167. Broekhuysen J, Degar F, Douchamps J, et al.: Pharmacokinetic study of cefuroxime in the elderly. Br J Clin Pharmacol 12:801–805
168. Kampmann J, Mølholm Hansen J, Siersback-Nielsen K, Laursen H: Effect of some drugs on penicillin half-life in blood. Clin Pharmacol Ther 13:516–519, 1972.
169. Leikola E, Vartia KO: On penicillin levels in young and geriatric subjects. J Gerontol 12:48–52, 1957.
170. Traeger A, Kiesewetter R, Kunge M: Zur Pharmakokinetik von Phenobarbital bei Erwachsenen und Greisen. Deutch Ges Wesen 29:1040–1042, 1974.
171. Castleden CM, Kaye CM, Parsons RL: The effect of age on plasma levels of propranolol and practolol in man. Br J Clin Pharmacol 2:303–306, 1975.
172. Kramer PA, Chapron DJ, Benson J, Mercik SA: Tetracycline absorption in elderly patients with achlorhydria. Clin Pharmacol Ther 23:467–472, 1978.
173. Vir SC, Love AHG: Nutritional status of institutionalized and noninstitutionalized aged in Belfast, Northern Ireland. Am J Clin Nutr 32:1934–1947, 1979.
174. Kohrs MB, O'Neal R, Preston A, et al.: Nutritional status of elderly residents in Missouri. Am J Clin Nutr 31:2186–2197, 1978.
175. Yearick ES, Wang MSL, Pisias SJ: Nutritional status of the elderly: Dietary and biochemical findings. J Gerontol 35:663–671, 1980.
176. Department of Health and Social Security, England. Rep Health Soc Subject No. 16, 1979.

5

Risks of Drug-Induced Hypercholesterolemia and Hypocholesterolemia in the Elderly

Daphne A. Roe

PLASMA LIPID AND LIPOPROTEIN LEVELS IN THE ELDERLY AND THE RISK OF CORONARY HEART DISEASE

In the first National Health and Nutrition Examination Survey (N-HANES I), there were 3,479 persons aged 65 to 74 years, corresponding to 12,773,000 in this age group in the total population.[1] Lowenstein[2] presented major findings on serum cholesterol values in this group of the population. These serum cholesterol values, separated by sex and race, are shown in Table 5-1. The higher mean serum cholesterol levels, which were observed in women aged 65–74 years, as compared with men of the same age group, are in accordance with previous findings that women past the menopause have cholesterol levels that surpass those of men after the age of 55.

Table 5-1. Serum Cholesterol Levels by Sex and Race of United States Individuals Aged 65 to 74 Years (HANES I, 1972–74)

Variable	White men	Black men	White women	Black women
Mean (mg/100 ml)	166.9 ± 30.8[a]	173.8 ± 32.2	180.0 ± 35.6[a]	185.3 ± 37.5
Percent below cutoff	<5%	<5%	<5%	<5%
Percent above cutoff	<5%	7%	12%	19%
Number	1,344	294	1,496	318
Serum cholesterol cutoff points: lowest = 120; highest = 220.				

[a] Significant at the .05 level of probability

Adapted from Lowenstein FW: Nutritional status of the elderly in the United States of America, 1971–1974. J Am Coll Nutr 1:169, 1982.

Pertinent to our present discussion is whether serum/plasma cholesterol levels indicate the risk of coronary artery disease events. Stamler,[3] in discussing the risk of a major coronary event (myocardial infarct) in relation to plasma cholesterol values, indicates that this risk increases with age even though the risk ratio relative to the cholesterol level is less in older men than in younger men. He states: "While the relative risk declines in older men, the attributable risk remains high and is an important guide for medical action."

Further information on plasma lipids and lipoprotein levels in the elderly is given in the reports of the Collaborative Lipid Research Clinics Program Prevalence Studies[4] and in the reports of the Cincinnati Lipid Research Clinic's studies.[5,6]

Glueck,[7] in describing the findings of his studies, focuses on the observation that both in men and women, plasma low-density lipoprotein cholesterol levels peak at about the sixth decade and then in the three subsequent decades fall abruptly. His interpretation is that the decline in the low-density lipoprotein cholesterol with age is probably explained by lethal myocardial infarction and stroke, which remove those people from the distribution having higher low-density lipoprotein cholesterol (C-LDL) levels. High-density lipoprotein cholesterol (C-HDL) levels after age 60 remain stable or rise moderately.

Whereas previously higher C-LDL levels were considered as a risk factor in atherosclerosis, in several studies reduced concentrations of C-HDL have been correlated with an increased susceptibility to coronary heart disease (CHD), with higher C-HDL levels having longer life expectancy and lower CHD mortality.[8,9,10]

ROLE OF CHANGE IN SMOKING HABITS, DIET, AND DRUGS IN THE DECLINE IN CORONARY ARTERY DISEASE MORTALITY

Levy, in discussing the decline in mortality from coronary artery disease since 1968, has evaluated the various possible explanations. He considers that the decline may be due both to improved patient care after acute heart attacks and also to risk factor modification. Within the category of risk factor modification, he includes decline in cigarette smoking. However, he is cautious about suggesting that the decline in coronary artery disease mortality is attributable to change in dietary pattern. Indeed, he suggests that it would be premature to associate decline in coronary artery disease mortality either with change in diet or with use of lipid-lowering drugs without first reviewing large-scale clinical trials of these modalities.

Therapeutic drugs may have influenced the mortality from heart disease, but this drug influence may run in both directions such that certain drugs may increase risk while others reduce risk. Such drugs as diuretics may elevate plasma cholesterol levels and cause a decline in plasma high-density lipoprotein levels.[12,13,14] Conversely, hypolipidemic drugs of the absorbable and nonabsorbable types may improve lipid status and decrease coronary risk but may impose nutritional or metabolic hazards.[15]

HYPERCHOLESTEROLEMIC EFFECTS OF DRUGS USED BY THE ELDERLY AND THE REVERSAL OF THESE EFFECTS

Thiazide Diuretics

Short- and long-term treatment of hypertension with thiazide diuretics has been shown to lead to increases in C-LDL and decreases in C-HDL levels. Cholesterol and plasma triglyceride levels may also be elevated.[14,16]

Thiazides may cause abnormalities of glucose as well as lipid metabolism, and the observed effects are similar to those occurring in maturity onset diabetes. In order to determine the reversibility of glucose intolerance associated with thiazide administration and to identify mechanisms responsible for alterations in carbohydrate and lipid metabolism associated with thiazide usage, Ames and Hill[17] examined the glucose tolerance test, insulin levels, glycosylated hemoglobin levels, and lipid concentrations of patients during the supervised withdrawal of long-term diuretic therapy. There were 35 patients in this study with primary hypertension. Glucose tolerance and glycosylated hemoglobin levels improved, and total cholesterol and triglyceride levels decreased seven weeks after cessation of the diuretic regime. The magnitude of change in lipid concentrations from the treated to the untreated state were correlated with changes in glycosylated hemoglobin. The suggestion was made by the investigators that insulin resistance develops during diuretic therapy, and it is the insulin resistance that causes the secondary disturbances in carbohydrate and lipid metabolism. In considering the implications of these findings for elderly populations in whom management of hypertension with thiazides is common practice, it is necessary to define the population at risk, examine the evidence of adverse health effects, and particularly effects on cardiovascular morbidity and mortality.

The Multiple Risk Factor Intervention Trial (MRFIT) showed that men in the intervention group who took thiazide diuretics (mostly hypertensives) had an elevation in plasma cholesterol and a diminished effect of diet in reducing hypercholesterolemia. A modest increase in plasma triglyceride levels was also observed. Analysis of the MRFIT data has also shown an association between electrocardiographic abnormalities, cardiovascular mortality, and high-dose thiazide therapy for hypertension. A suggestion has been made that the toxic effects of thiazides on the heart might be explained by drug-induced potassium deficiency on a previously damaged myocardium. However, this hypothesis has not been examined, nor is it known whether the effects of thiazides on lipid metabolism contribute to cardiac pathology.[18,19]

In considering the implications of the findings of the MRFIT study for elderly people in whom management of hypertension and avoidance of stroke are primary considerations, it is necessary to develop a screening procedure to identify those who are at high risk for the development of thiazide-related disorders of carbohydrate and lipid metabolism. From the findings of Ames and Hill, it would appear that the measurement of glycosylated hemoglobin levels may be an appropriate test. Individuals having elevated glycohemoglobin levels would be given alternate antihypertensive therapy.

An alternate approach to the problem of thiazide-related hyperlipoproteinemia has been proposed by Schiffl et al.[20] These authors showed that increases in serum low-density lipoprotein cholesterol, related to use of a thiazide diuretic, could be controlled by concurrent administration of a beta blocker. They showed that low doses of the thiazide clopamide combined with the beta blocker pindolol could offer effective treatment for moderate essential hypertension. The drugs were well tolerated, and it was shown that this combination treatment could be used to avoid the increase in serum C-LDL levels that occurs when clopamide is given alone.

Beta Blockers

The beta blocker propranolol is known to affect lipoprotein composition through its effects on fatty acids derived from adipose tissue and through its effects on lipid synthesis in the liver.[21,22] Since propranolol is an effective beta-adrenergic blocking drug that is widely used in the treatment of angina pectoris, hypertension, and various arrhythmias that occur in the elderly and that are usually associated with atherosclerosis, it is important to define long-term effects of this drug on lipid metabolism.

The long-term effects of propranolol on plasma lipids and lipoprotein composition were investigated by Tanaka et al.[23] The subjects were five men and five postmenopausal women of 48–79 years of age resident in Japan. They had all had several vascular accidents more than six months before the period of observation. Subjects were given the regular hospital diet, which consisted of 2,200 calories, of which 60% were from carbohydrate (55% from starch, 5% from sugar), 17% from protein, and 23% from fat. Determinations were made of blood glucose, immunoreactive insulin, total lipids, free fatty acids, triglyceride levels, total and free cholesterol levels, and phospholipids, as well as plasma lipoprotein levels. No significant changes in caloric intake, diet composition, body weight, blood glucose, or circulating plasma volume were seen during the study. Immunoreactive insulin levels were slightly decreased in four patients but were stable in the others. Plasma-free fatty acids began to increase after a slight decrease in the first week of propranolol treatment, whereas triglyceride levels and total cholesterol were not significantly affected by the drug. Both free-cholesterol and phospholipid levels were decreased approximately 15% by the eighth week of treatment. There was an increase in lipids of the very low density lipoprotein class, and a decrease in lipids of both low- and high-density lipoproteins.

In a study reported by Bauer et al.,[24] it was found that when propranolol was used as an adjunct to antihypertensive therapy using a thiazide diuretic, the beta blocker caused an increase in very low density lipoprotein levels, especially in subjects receiving hydrochlorothiazide. In this study, propranolol alone had no effect on plasma lipid levels.

A cross-section and longitudinal study was carried out that involved 1,462 women of five strata (aged 38–60 years at the beginning of the study) resident in Göteborg, Sweden. Initial study of these women was from 1968–1969, and there was a restudy from 1974 to 1975. Women taking thiazide diuretics and beta blockers were identified and followed up. In the cross-sectional study, it was shown that the women receiving beta blockers had increased serum triglyceride levels. This relationship was also shown in the longitudinal study. Interestingly, in this study no significant changes in carbohydrate or lipid metabolism were found in women receiving thiazide diuretics.[25] A question that still remains unanswered is the extent to which the lipid composition of the diet affects the impact of thiazides and of beta blockers, such as propranolol, on lipid status.

USE AND ABUSE OF HYPOCHOLESTEROLEMIC DRUGS IN THE ELDERLY

Elderly patients with atherosclerotic cardiovascular or cerebrovascular disease are frequently prescribed hypocholesterolemic agents, particularly when hypercholesterolemia is marked. Further, hypocholesterolemic agents may be taken by elderly patients for other medical problems. For example, niacin may be taken as a cerebral vasodilator, cholestyramine may be given as a means to correct for oxaluria secondary to ileal disease or resection, and neomycin may be used in the management of incipient liver failure associated with cirrhosis.[26,27,28] In the elderly, it is particulary important to consider the nutritional and metabolic side effects of these drugs since the side effects may be of more consequence than the therapeutic value of the drugs.

Niacin

The hypocholesterolemic effects of large doses of niacin were first reported by Altschul et al. In 1955.[29] Since that time, niacin has been in use as a hypocholesterolemic agent, and although use of niacin as a hypocholestcrolcmic drug declined after the mid-1960s for several years, now again it is used as an adjunct drug with a bile acid sequestrant. Niacin may be prescribed for elderly patients with elevated serum cholesterol levels who also have evidence of cerebrovascular disease. The rationale for such treatment is that niacin is both a hypocholesterolemic agent and a vasodilator. In fact, however, there is no evidence of sustained vasodilatation associated with administration of niacin in pharmacological doses.[30]

It has been demonstrated that niacin decreases total plasma triglycerides and very low density lipoprotein triglyceride. It also decreases plasma cholesterol and increases the hepatic secretion of biliary cholesterol.[31]

Reported side effects occurring in patients receiving niacin therapy at dosages $\geqslant$300 mg per day include flushing, dryness of the skin, nausea and diarrhea, and, rarely, the skin changes of acanthosis nigricans. Some patients have developed impaired hepatic function, hyperglycemia, and hyperuricemia. Hepatotoxicity with elevation of plasma transaminases and alkaline phosphatase is dose dependent, occurring with greater frequency when the niacin dose exceeds 2.5 g per month. Glucose intolerance is usually moderate. Hyperuricemia occurs in about one third of the patients receiving pharmacological doses of niacin but is not usually associated with gout. Arrhythmia has been described.

Whereas the prostaglandin-mediated vasodilator effects of niacin, including the flushing and infrequently associated tachycardia, tinnitis, and pruritus, may be partially or completely inhibited by aspirin (0.3 g), the hepatotoxic and other metabolic effects of niacin can only be reversed when the "drug" is discontinued.[32,33,34]

Glueck,[35] in describing the side effects of niacin, mentions gastritis, esophagitis, and duodenal ulcer. He is of the opinion that a careful watch should be made for the appearance of these complications and if upper GI symptoms occur, niacin treatment should be discontinued.

Considering, then, that niacin given in pharmacological doses has the capacity not only to induce unpleasant but also health-threatening side effects, the question arises whether it is ever justifiable to give it to elderly patients who are at risk for events related to atherosclerotic heart disease or cerebrovascular episodes (transient ischemia and stroke). We know that high doses of niacin elevate high-density lipoprotein levels and that higher HDL values are associated with a lower risk of coronary disease. However, as pointed out by Rodstein,[36] although niacin ingestion is correlated with higher HDL levels, there is no proof that in altering HDL levels in the elderly there is a beneficial effect such that the mortality from atherosclerotic disease is reduced.

Bile Acid Sequestrants

In young and middle-aged people with hyperlipoproteinemias of the type II, type III, and type IV groups, the risk of premature death from myocardial infarct is excessively high, and usually drug treatment is with a bile acid sequestrant with or without added niacin. The bile acid sequestrants that are used include cholestyramine and colestipol. These anionic resins bind bile acids in the intestine and potentiate fecal excretion. The production of bile acids from cholesterol is increased. The pools of cholesterol are decreased during therapy with these bile acid-binding resins, and the content of cholesteryl esters in low-density lipoprotein particles is somewhat decreased.[37,38]

In the past, the adverse nutritional side effects of cholestyramine and colestipol have been emphasized. High doses of cholestyramine cause malabsorption of fat-soluble vitamins, particularly vitamins A and K, because of the drug-induced lack of bile acids for their absorption. Reports of steatorrhea and of deficiencies of fat-soluble vitamins relate to individuals taking doses of the resin in excess of 16 g/day or to individuals with preexisting bile disease.[39,40,41]

West and Lloyd[42] have shown that with long-time use of cholestyramine, folacin depletion may develop. Cholestyramine has also been reported to impair absorption of vitamin B_{12}.[43]

Long-term effects of colestipol on serum concentrations of fat-soluble vitamins have been studied, and it has been shown that serum levels of vitamins A and E may decrease over time. However, in evaluating these findings, it is important to note that the studies were carried out in children, and that the children were on low-cholesterol diets. No clinical evidence of vitamin A or vitamin E deficiency was observed.[44]

Drug/drug interactions, rather than drug/nutrient interactions, are the major hazard of administering cholestyramine or colestipol to the elderly. These resins can bind a number of drugs and interfere with their absorption. The drugs bound by this resin include those taken commonly by older people, including digitalis glycosides, warfarin, thiazide diuretics, tetracycline, phenobarbital, and thyroxine. There is a likelihood that one or more of these drugs could be taken concurrently with cholestyramine or colestipol because of multiple health problems. It is important that the drug in question be given at least one hour, and preferably two hours, before the resin.[34]

The most frequent side effect of cholestyramine and colestipol is constipation, which, however, even in the elderly, can usually be treated by the addition of bran cereal to the diet.

COMBINED THERAPIES OF HETEROZYGOUS FAMILIAL HYPERCHOLESTEROLEMIA WITH A BILE ACID SEQUESTRANT AND NIACIN

In heterozygous familial hypercholesterolemia, circulating low-density lipoprotein levels are two to three times the normal range, and high-affinity receptors for LDL and cell membranes are deficient.[45,46] Knowledge of the specific aberrations of lipid transport and disposition in familial hypercholesterolemia has focused interest on the need to use therapeutic regimens that not only reduce serum cholesterol but also decrease plasma C-LDL.

Kane et al.[47] compared the effects of diet alone, colestipol alone, colestipol with clofibrate, and colestipol with niacin in 50 people who all met the diagnostic criteria for heterozygous familial hypercholesterolemia. Particular interests of this study are that there were 21 men and 29 women who spanned the ages of 19–71 years. Thirty-seven of the patients had tendinous xanthomata. All patients included in the study were given a diet low in cholesterol and saturated fats. In patients who were to receive 20 gm of colestipol per day, serum cholesterol levels fell by an average of 16% during the period prior to the initiation of drug therapy. Then there was a further decrease of 16%–25% in serum cholesterol during a year on colestipol. Addition of clofibrate produced a total mean decrease in serum cholesterol of 28%. When colestipol was given in combination with niacin, low-density lipoprotein cholesterol decreased 55%. Tendinous xanthomata were significantly reduced in size by this combination regime.

Observed side effects included constipation in patients on colestipol alone, and elevation in serum creatine phosphokinase activity in patients taking clofibrate. Patients on niacin showed transient abnormalities in liver function tests when the dose was increased rapidly. While taking colestipol and niacin, 4 patients out of the 22 taking this combination had mild gastric irritation. One patient on niacin had a dermatosis that necessitated discontinuation of therapy. Most patients on niacin experienced flushing at the beginning of the treatment period.[47] The authors concluded that colestipol plus niacin may be useful in the treatment of patients "at high risk from elevated levels of LDL."

RISKS OF TREATING RISK FACTORS

The risk of treating risk factors for one disease with drugs is the chemical induction of a new risk factor for the same disease or for a different disease. Thiazides are effective in the management of mild to moderate hypertension. However, thiazide-induced glucose intolerance and hypercholesterolemia may be risk factors for cardiovascular morbidity and mortality. Stamler,[3] in stressing the need for primary prevention of hypertension, wrote: "Medical practitioners and public health physicians cannot be satisfied with mass prescription of drugs for years on end as the main means of hypertension control. . . . In the elderly, hypertensive measures are therapeutic rather than prophylactic, unless with the term *prophylaxis* the prevention of cerebrovascular accidents is included." Present research needs are not only to identify patients who have characteristics that place them at risk for the development of hyperglycemia and hypercholesterolemia, but also to further evaluate antihypertensive therapies that diminish or obviate these risks.

Whether to treat hypercholesterolemia or other lipid disorders that confer an increased risk of coronary heart disease may be an age-related decision. The short-term nutritional and metabolic side effects of hypolipidemic agents should certainly make physicians reflect on the wisdom of such treatment, especially when there is limited evidence of benefit in relation to cardiovascular morbidity or mortality of older individuals. Further, the wisdom of using hypocholesterolemic agents has been placed in doubt by findings of an inverse association between serum cholesterol and cancer in males. This inverse association has been found to be significant in relation to colon cancer, and it is more apparent at older ages. From the point of view of nutrition and cancer, it is interesting and may be important to note that individuals with low plasma cholesterol values may also have low plasma retinol values.[48] Lower plasma retinol values have been associated with an increased risk of lung and gastrointestinal cancer.[49,50]

It has also been suggested that an excessive amount of bile acids in the feces may promote colon cancer.[5] Increased fecal bile acids and decreased absorption of beta carotene and retinol are well recognized as outcomes of cholestyramine and colestipol therapy. These observations place in doubt the wisdom of administering bile acid sequestrants to people in age groups in which there is a high incidence of cancer, particularly lung and gastrointestinal cancer. Indeed, panelists at the May 1981 Workshop on Cholesterol and Noncardiovascular Disease Mortality, jointly sponsored by the National Heart and Lung and Blood Institute and the National Cancer Institute, recognized a need for research "on bile acids and dietary lipids in relation to the absorption of vitamin A."[48]

In view of the current state of ignorance about the long-term effects of drug-induced nutritional and metabolic disorders, there is an urgent need for well-designed case control studies of cardiovascular and neoplastic disease in individuals who have received chronic therapy with hypolipemic, as well as hypotensive, agents and in appropriate controls.

REFERENCES

1. United States Department of Health, Education and Welfare: Total serum cholesterol levels of adults 18–74 years, United States, 1971–74. DHEW Publication No. (PHS)78-1652, Series 11, No. 205. Hyattsville, Md, USDHEW/PHS, National Center for Health Statistics, April 1978.
2. Lowenstein FW: Nutritional status of the elderly in the United States of America, 1971–1974. J Am Coll Nutr 1:165–177, 1982.
3. Stamler J: Disease of the cardiovascular system. In Clark D.W, MacMahon B (eds): Preventive and Community Medicine. 2nd ed. Boston, Little, Brown, 1981, pp 193–217.
4. Circulation: High-density lipoprotein cholesterol: The Lipid Research Clinics Program Prevalence Study. Circulation 62 (suppl 4), 1980.
5. Laskarzewski P, Morrison JA, Horvitz R, et al.: The relationship of parental history of myocardial infarction, hypertension, diabetes, and stroke to coronary heart disease factors in their adult progeny. Am J Epidemiol 113:290–307, 1981.
6. Gartside PS, Morrison JA, Kahoury P, et al.: Clustering and interrelationships of high, low, and very low density lipoproteins in hypolipidemic children and adults: Cincinnati Lipid Research Clinic, Princeton School Prevalence Study. Prev Med 10:1–14, 1981.
7. Glueck CJ: Cradle-to-grave atherosclerosis: High-density lipoprotein cholesterol. J Am Coll Nutr 1:41–48, 1982.
8. Philip Eaton R, Allan RC Jr, Koopmans LH, et al.: Overview of lipoprotein metabolism. Perspectives in a free-living southwest population in Bernalillo County, New Mexico. In Garry PJ (ed): Human Nutrition: Clinical and Biochemical Aspects. Proceedings of the Fourth Arnold O. Beckman Conf, Clin Chem Washington, Assoc Clin Chem, 1980, pp 109–131.
9. Glueck CJ, Fallat RW, Millett F, et al.: Familial hyperalpha-lipoproteinemia: Studies in 18 kindreds. Metabolism 24:1234–1265, 1975.

10. Glueck CJ, Gartside PS, Steiner PM, et al.: Hyperalpha- and hyperbeta-lipoproteinemia in octogenarian kindreds. Atherosclerosis 27:387–406, 1977.
11. Levy RI. The decline in cardiovascular disease mortality. Ann Rev Pub Hlth 2:49–70, 1981.
12. Schoenfeld MR, Goldberger E. Hypercholesterolemia induced by thiazides: A pilot study. Curr Ther Res 6:180, 1964.
13. Johnson B, Bye C, Labrooy I, et al.: The relation of antihypertensive treatment to plasma lipids and other vascular risk factors in hypertension. Clin Sci Mol Med 47:9, 1974.
14. Grimm RH Jr, Leon AS, Hunninghake DB, et al.: Effects of thiazide diuretics on plasma lipids and lipoproteins in mildly hypertensive patients. A double-blind control trial. Ann Intern Med 94:7–11, 1981.
15. Miettinen TA: Effects of hypolipidemic drugs on bile acid metabolism in man. Adv Lipid Res 18:65–97, 1981.
16. Joos C, Kewitz H, Reinhold-Kouniati D: Effects of diuretics on plasma lipoproteins in healthy men. Eur J Clin Pharmacol 17:251–257, 1980.
17. Ames RP, Hill P: Improvement of glucose tolerance and lowering of glycohemoglobin and serum lipid concentrations after discontinuation of antihypertensive drug therapy. Circulation 65:899–904, 1982.
18. Multiple Risk Factor Intervention Trial Research Group: Multiple Risk Factor Intervention Trial: Risk factor changes and mortality results. JAMA 248:1465–1477, 1982.
19. Editorial: A heart study produces a surprise result. Science 218:31–32, 1982.
20. Schiffl H, Weidmann P, Mordasini R, et al.: Reversal of diuretic-induced increases in serum low-density-lipoprotein cholesterol by the beta blocker pindolol. Metabolism 31:411–415, 1982.
21. Imura H, Ikeda M, Morimoto M, Yawata M: Effect of adrenergic blocking or stimulating agents in plasma growth hormone, immunoreactive insulin, and blood free fatty acid levels in man. J Clin Invest 50:1069–1079, 1971.
22. Barboliak JJ, Friedberg HD: Propranolol and hypertriglyceridemia. Atherosclerosis 17:31–33, 1973.
23. Tanaka N, Sakaguchi S, Oshige K, et al.: Effect of chronic administration of propranolol on lipoprotein composition. Metabolism 25:1071–1075, 1976.
24. Bauer JH, Brooks CS, Weinstein I, et al.: Effects of diuretic and propranolol on plasma lipoprotein lipids. Clin Pharmacol Therap 30:35–43, 1981.
25. Bengtsson C, Lennartsson J, Lindquist O, et al.: On the metabolic effects of diuretics and beta blockers. Results from a cross-sectional and longitudinal population study of women. Acta Med Scand 212:57–64, 1982.
26. Nickerson M: Vasodilator drugs. In Goodman LS, Gilman A (eds): The Pharmacological Basis of Therapeutics, 5th ed. New York, Macmillan, 1975, pp 736–737.
27. Isselbacher KJ: Malabsorption syndromes including disease of pancreatic and biliary origin. In Winick M (ed): Nutrition and Gastroenterology. New York, Wiley, 1980, pp 101–103.
28. Faloon WW: Drug production of intestinal malabsorption. NY State J Med 70:2189–2191, 1970.
29. Altschul R, Hoffer A, Stephen JD: Influence of nicotinic acid on serum cholesterol in man. Arch Biochem Biophys 54:558–559, 1955.
30. Cook P, James I: Cerebral vasodilators. 2. New Engl J Med 305:1560–1564, 1981.
31. Grundy SM, Mok HYI, Zec L, Berman M: Influence of nicotinic acid on metabolism of cholesterol and triglycerides in man. J Lipid Res 22:24–36, 1981.

32. Kuo PT, Kostis JB, Moreyra AE, Hayes JA: Familial type II hyperlipoproteinemia with coronary heart disease: Effect of diet-colestipol-nicotinic acid treatment. Chest 79:286–291, 1981.
33. Illingworth DR, Phillipson BE, Rapp JH, Connor WE: Colestipol plus nicotinic acid in treatment of heterozygous familial hypercholesterolaemia. Lancet 1:296–298, 1981.
34. Havel RJ, Kane JP: Therapy of hyperlipidemic states. Ann Rev Med 33:417–433, 1982.
35. Glueck CJ: Colestipol and probucol: Treatment of primary and familial hypercholesterolemia and amelioration of atherosclerosis. Ann Intern Med 96:475–482, 1982.
36. Rodstein M: Ischemic and hypertensive heart disease in the aged: Prognostic and therapeutic factors. J Am Geriat Soc 35:388–395, 1980.
37. Moutafis CD, Simson LA, Myant NB, et al.: The effect of cholestyramine on the faecal excretion of bile acids and neutral steroids in familial hypercholesterolaemia. Atherosclerosis 26:329–334, 1977.
38. Grundy SM, Mok HYI: Colestipol, clofibrate, and phytosterols in combined therapy of hyperlipidemia. J Lab Clin Med 89:354–366, 1977.
39. Heaton KW, Lever JV, Barnard D. Osteomalacia associated with cholestyramine therapy for post-iliectomy diarrhea. Gastroenterology 62:642–646, 1972.
40. Gross L, Brotman M: Hypoprothrombinemia and hemorrhage associated with cholestyramine therapy. Ann Intern Med 72:95–96, 1970.
41. Roe DA: Drug-Induced Nutritional Deficiencies. Westport, Conn, AVI Publishing, 1976.
42. West RJ, Lloyd JK: The effect of cholestyramine on intestinal absorption. Gut 16:93–98, 1975.
43. Coronato A, Glass GBJ: Depression of the intestinal uptake of radiovitamin B-12 by cholestyramine. Proc Soc Exp Biol Med 142:1341–1344, 1973.
44. Schwarz KB, Goldstein PD, Witztum JL, Schoenfeld G: Fat-soluble vitamin concentrations in hypercholesterolemic children treated with colestipol. Pediatrics 65:243–250, 1980.
45. Goldstein JL, Brown MS: Familial hypercholesterolemia: A genetic regulatory defect in cholesterol metabolism. Am J Med 58:147–150, 1975.
46. Goldstein J, Brown MS: The low-density lipoprotein pathway and its relationship to atherosclerosis. Ann Rev Biochem 46:897–940, 1977.
47. Kane JP, Malloy MJ, Tun P, et al.: Normalization of low-density-lipoprotein levels in heterozygous familial hypercholesterolemia with a combined drug regimen. New Engl J Med 304:251–258, 1981.
48. Feinlieb M: Summary of workshop on cholesterol and noncardiovascular disease mortality. Prev Med 11:360–367, 1982.
49. Wald N, Idle M, Boreham J: Low serum–vitamin A and subsequent risk of cancer. Lancet 2:813–815, 1980.
50. Mettlin C, Graham S, Swanson M: Vitamin A and lung cancer. J Nat Cancer Inst 62:1435–1438, 1979.
51. Reddy BS: Nutrition and colon cancer. In Draper HH (ed): Advances in Nutrition Research, vol. 2. New York, Plenum Press, 1979, pp 199–218.

6 | Drug-Induced Mineral Depletion in the Elderly

Daphne A. Roe

MULTIFACTORIAL ETIOLOGY OF MINERAL DEPLETION

Drug-induced mineral depletion in the elderly is largely explained by their pattern of drug usage. In a British study in which physicians to geriatric medicine departments were asked to make returns on drug usage by patients being admitted to their extended care facilities, it was shown that prescription drugs that were being taken by more than 10% of the total sample included diuretics, analgesics, antidepressants and tranquilizers, sedatives, digitalis, and potassium salts, as well as antibiotics and antibacterials. Laxatives, vasodilators, bronchodilators, and rigidity- or tremor-controlling drugs were taken by more than 5% of this population. Diuretics were easily the most widely prescribed drugs, followed by analgesics, psychotropic agents, and digitalis.[1]

In a review of the United States experience of drugs taken by the elderly, Ouslander[2] reported that cardiovascular drugs (digitalis, diuretics, antihypertensives), psychotropic drugs (sedatives, hypnotics, antipsychotics), analgesics, and laxatives were the most frequently prescribed.

Within the drug groups commonly taken by the elderly, there are many that cause mineral depletion. For example, the most common drugs causing potassium deficiency are diuretics, both of the thiazide and loop types. In the elderly who have several concurrent chronic diseases, as well as health complaints for which they seek palliative relief, it is not uncommon for patients to be taking several drugs at the same time that can cause mineral deficiencies. Thus, intake of thiazide diuretics and laxatives can have an additive effect on potassium losses, or concurrent intake of aminoglycoside and cephalosporin antibiotics can have an interactive effect that induces mineral depletion, with large renal losses of potassium and magnesium.

Clinical investigations have indicated that responses to many drugs change as people age. This is indeed true of drugs that induce mineral depletion. It is generally accepted that the elderly are more susceptible to mineral depletion related to drug intake because of multiple drug usage, but also because of prolonged drug intake. When a drug causes a mild hyperexcretion of a specific mineral, over time a mineral deficiency may develop and induce symptoms. Further, physiological changes related to aging may also predispose to drug-related mineral depletion.

Crooks and Stevenson[3] brought to our attention once again the relationship between an age-related decline in renal function and potential for mineral depletion by nephrotoxic drugs. When drugs are excreted by simple glomerular filtration, their rate of excretion decreases with glomerular filtration rate and hence with creatinine clearance. Slowed rate of elimination of digoxin and the aminoglycoside antibiotics by the elderly may be related to the decline in renal function, though with these antibiotics another factor is the primary nephrotoxicity of the drug.[4]

Skeletal muscles, bone, and most other tissues of the body demonstrate that with age there is a physical loss of tissue mass varying in amount from 7% to 30%. Mineral depletion occurs with loss of lean body mass. This loss, which is age-related, may influence the development of mineral deficiency with drug intake.[5] Age-related diseases can potentiate drug-related mineral depletion in the elderly, more particularly renal disease and catabolic diseases, including metastatic cancer.[6,7]

Alcohol-related diseases, including cirrhosis, which are not uncommon in the elderly, may also contribute to mineral depletion. In alcoholics, losses of potassium, calcium, magnesium, and zinc are increased.[8]

Elderly people may also have inadequate dietary intakes of potassium, calcium, magnesium, and zinc. However, it was pointed out by Exton-Smith and Overstall[9] that inadequate nutrient intake, including mineral intake, is related to low food energy intake. Low nutrient intake by elderly people was explained in Exton-Smith's survey subjects either by late effects of partial or total gastrectomy, or by the presence of chronic disabling physical disease or depression.[10]

This chapter examines drug causes of specific mineral depletions and describes the clinical and biochemical features of drug-related mineral depletion in the elderly. Under the umbrella term *drug-induced mineral depletion,* particular conditions are included that lead to a decline in the plasma level of the particular mineral and also those in which there is an actual tissue depletion.

SODIUM

Distribution and Function

Sodium is the most abundant cation of those found in the extracellular fluid. It is essential to the regulation of the acid/base balance and is a very important contributor to extracellular osmolality. It functions in the electrophysiology of cells and is required for the propagation of impulses in excitable tissues. Sodium is also essential for active nutrient transport, including the active transport of glucose across the intestinal musoca.[11]

Hyponatremia

Common mechanisms responsible for hyponatremia include (1) increase in body water (usually known as dilutional hyponatremia); (2) decrease in body solute (net sodium loss); and (3) addition of solute to plasma, causing an osmotic redistribution of water.[12]

Drugs Causing Sodium Depletion

Arieff et al.[13] have discussed the neurological and non-neurological signs of hyponatremia and sodium depletion. Acute hyponatremia, when severe, is associated with depression of the sensorium, and patients may have grand mal seizures. Common symptoms include anorexia, nausea, vomiting, and muscle weakness. In the elderly, symptoms of sodium depletion may be attributed to debility, potassium deficiency, or digitalis intoxication. Drugs causing hyponatremia and sodium depletion are shown in Table 6-1.

Drug-induced hyponatremia and sodium depletion treatment requires stopping the responsible drug. Water restriction is required when drug-related syndrome of inappropriate antidiuretic hormone secretion (SIADH) has induced water intoxication. Further, in symptomatic cases of hyponatremia, hypertonic saline may need to be administered to diminish the risk of fatal brain edema.[14]

Drugs can cause all three types of hyponatremia. Drug-induced dilutional hyponatremia is due to the production of SIADH.[15]

Several drug groups commonly taken by the elderly have an antidiuretic action. Among these are the oral hypoglycemic agents, including chlorpropamide, which has been shown to have an antidiuretic effect in patients with diabetes insipidus and also in patients with diabetes mellitus. Tolbutamide has also been reported as a cause of a similar type of dilutional hyponatremia.[16,17]

It has been pointed out by Weissman et al.[18] that chlorpropamide-induced hyponatremia is more frequently found in patients who have a tendency to retain fluid, such as those with congestive heart failure or cirrhosis.[18] The more frequent occurrence of chlorpropamide-induced hyponatremia in older patients is due to the

Table 6-1. Common Drugs Causing Dilutional Hyponatremia and Sodium Depletion in the Elderly

Dilutional Hyponatremia	Hyponatremia with Sodium Depletion
Chlorpropamide	Thiazides
Tolbutamide	Spironolactone
Vincristine	Captopril
Amitryptyline	
Mannitol	

extensive use of this oral hypoglycemic agent to treat older maturity-onset diabetics and the prevalence of congestive heart failure within this population.

Two cancer chemotherapeutic agents have been shown to produce SIADH. Vincristine usually causes water retention within one to two weeks after the beginning of treatment.[19] Cyclophosphamide can produce its antidiuretic effect beginning about 4–12 hours after injection and lasting for up to 20 hours.[20]

Two tricyclic drugs, carbamazepine and amitryptyline, have been reported to produce SIADH.[21,22] Because of the common use of amitryptyline as an antidepressant in the elderly, the risk of hyponatremia should not be overlooked.

Hyponatremia from sodium depletion may occur with diuretic therapy. Thiazides have been reported as the cause of serious and fatal hyponatremia in elderly patients. Hyponatremia occurring with thiazide administation develops rather slowly and will usually resolve rapidly when the drug is discontinued, unless the patient has been drinking very large volumes of water.[23]

The aldosterone antagonist spironolactone may cause hyponatremia because the body's capacity to conserve sodium is temporarily lost.[24] Hyponatremia following administration of captopril has also been reported, and it has been suggested that this drug also produces hyponatremia and sodium depletion because of an antialdosterone effect. The five men with captopril-induced hyponatremia reported by Nicholls et al.[25] were between the ages of 54 and 72 years, and all had congestive heart failure. Plasma sodium concentrations fell when the captopril was used to treat resistant heart failure, and then there was a parallel decline in circulating concentrations of angiotensin II and aldosterone, and reciprocal elevation in plasma renin activity and plasma potassium concentration.

Hyponatremia is quite often observed during mannitol infusions. Infused mannitol molecules remain within the plasma compartment and raise the plasma osmolality. Water enters the extracellular space from cells until an osmotic balance is regained. The outcome is that there is a reduction in cell volume with concomitant expansion of circulating plasma volume and a lowering of plasma sodium concentration.[11] Flear and Singh[26] developed the concept of an association between hyponatremia and "sick cells." In seriously ill patients, the ability of cell membranes to retain organic solutes may be impaired, and the solutes may escape into the extracellular fluid in a manner analogous to that occurring when mannitol is infused. This condition in which isoosmotic redistribution of water follows has been called the "sick cell syndrome" and is also associated with hyponatremia.[27]

In cancer patients, hyponatremia may be the result of ectopic synthesis of antidiuretic hormone by the tumor tissue or excessive release of ADH from the neurohypophysis. However, hyponatremia in cancer patients can also have a dual or mixed etiology. Contributing factors include cancer chemotherapeutic drugs, such as vincristine and cyclophosphamide, and mannitol used to hydrate patients and diminish the risk of nephrotoxicity prior to cisplatin administration.[28,29]

Whereas it has been reported by Trump[30] that hyponatremia due to inappropriate ADH secretion of tumor origin can be treated in cancer patients by administration of demeclocycline, which is an ADH antagonist, this drug may have a nephrotoxic effect in cancer patients, and if the hyponatremia is not due to SIADH, then the drug will be ineffective.

POTASSIUM

Functions

Potassium has four major biological functions. It contributes to the maintenance of electrolyte balance, the transmission of nerve impulses to muscle fibers, the control of normal muscle contractility, and the control of heart rhythm. Potassium also acts as an insulin antagonist in intermediary carbohydrate metabolism.

Potassium Deficiency

Potassium deficiency and hypokalemia are certainly not synonymous. Nardone et al.[31] have estimated that approximately 98% of total body potassium is contained in the intracellular compartment of the body, and less than 2% is located in the serum, where it can be extracted for measurement. However, low serum or plasma potassium levels usually reflect total body deficits. In alkalosis due to insulin therapy or hypoosmolality, however, there may be a decrease in serum levels of potassium without a concomitant decrease in cellular potassium so that plasma potassium levels do not then actually reflect body stores.

Symptoms of potassium deficiency are weakness, anorexia, nausea, vomiting, listlessness, apprehension, and diffuse pain that is not always present. Drowsiness, stupor, and irrationality also develop with more serious degrees of potassium deficiency. Polydipsia and polyuria may occur with potassium deficiency due to renal tubular damage. Most prominent among the characteristic signs of potassium deficiency are cardiac arrhythmias, including atrial fibrillation, and in patients who have had myocardial infarcts, potassium deficiency is a major risk factor for the development of ventricular fibrillation.[32,33]

Drugs Causing Potassium Depletion

Hypokalemia with potassium depletion has been recognized as a potentially serious side effect of oral diuretic therapy. Diuretic drugs causing hypokalemia include thiazides and the loop diuretics furosemide and ethacrynic acid.[34,35]

Steen[32] has sown doubt on the contribution of low potassium intake to the development of hypokalemia in British patients receiving diuretics. However, elderly patients may consume diets that are low in potassium because of an inadequate intake of fruits and vegetables. An associated shortcoming of such diets is that they are low in dietary fiber, which may favor the development of constipation and hence laxative abuse.

Hypokalemia is also associated with laxative abuse because of loss of potassium into the gastrointestinal tract and failure of potassium reabsorption from the colon. Patients who have chronic and excessive intakes of phenolphthalein, bisacodyl, and senna have been reported with severe hypokalemia for which the cause was not discovered until their laxative abusive habits were suspected and/or proved.[36,37]

Hypokalemia may occur in the elderly, as in younger age groups, during prolonged high dosage of corticosteroid therapy. Corticosteroid-induced hypokalemia occurs with intake of natural and synthetic corticosteroids that have mineralocorticoid activity, and also with corticosteroids that have greater metabolic effect. Potassium is mobilized from tissues and excreted in the urine.[38]

Hypokalemic, hypochloremic alkalosis can develop with corticosteroids administration. It is our experience that in the elderly, hypokalemia is most likely to develop in patients with polymyositis and/or dermatomyositis who are receiving high-dosage corticosteroid therapy as treatment for profoundly catabolic diseases. Hypokalemia related to the use of potassium-losing diuretics is exacerbated by administration of corticosteroids.[39]

High or massive intake of salicylates can also produce hypokalemia. Salicylate hypokalemia is due to leakage of potassium from cells and also from the direct toxic effect of the drug on the kidney.[40]

Hypokalemia can occur with administration of antibiotics that have nephrotoxic potential. Included are gentamicin and amphotericin B.[41,42] O'Brien et al.[43] described an elderly female patient in whom hypokalemia developed after she took an overdose of the beta-adrenergic antagonist solbutamol. This drug, in common with catecholamines and other sympathomimetic agents, causes transfer of potassium from the extracellular to the intracellular compartments by activating sodium/potassium-dependent adenosine triphosphatase (ATPase). Hypokalemia has previously been described when the drug was given intravenously to insulin-dependent and nondependent diabetics.[44]

Hypokalemia, which is sometimes severe, has been reported in certain patients with parkinsonism who have been treated with levodopa. The influence of levodopa on the renal excretion of potassium was studied by Granerus et al.[45] in three patients with hypokalemia and in five normokalemic patients. Levodopa intake was found to cause an increase in potassium excretion in the hypokalemic, but not in the normokalemic, patients. This effect of levodopa was inhibited by the administration of a dopa decarboxylase inhibitor. It is not clear why hyperkaliuria occurs in some patients receiving levodopa and not in others.

Special Problems of Drug-Induced Potassium Deficiency in the Elderly

Diuretics and digitalis are the core drugs for elderly patients with heart disease, with or without congestive heart failure. Steiness,[46] in discussing the etiology of digitalis toxicity, has commented that both diuretic-induced hypokalemia and digitalis inhibit membrane sodium/potassium ATPase activity, which then causes a decrease in the intracellular potassium concentration. Risk of cardiac arrythmias during digitalis treatment and also during severe hypokalemia may explain in part additive effects of hypokalemia and digitalis on the myocardium. The myocardial uptake of digitalis is increased at low extracellular potassium concentrations, which may also in part explain the interactive effects between digitalis and hypokalemia. Further, the myocardial digoxin kinetic is changed during hypokalemia, but the renal excretion rate of digitalis is reduced at the same time, leading to increased serum digoxin concentration, which increases the risk of digitalis intoxication.

Table 6-2. Common Drugs Causing Hypokalemia and Potassium Depletion in the Elderly

Thiazides
Furosemide
Ethacrynic acid
Phenolphthalein
Bisacodyl
Senna
Corticosteroids
Salicylates (toxic dose)
Gentamicin
Amphotericin B
Levodopa

In the elderly, potassium depletion is frequently multifactorial. Contributory factors include low potassium intake from the diet and intake of several drugs, including diuretics, laxatives, and levodopa, which can singly or together produce hypokalemia and potassium deficiency.[36,47] Elderly patients who have the habit of taking excessive amounts of diuretics and laxatives are commonly those with obsessional disorders.[48]

Drugs causing potassium depletion in the elderly are shown in Table 6-2.

CALCIUM

Distribution and Function

Calcium is the most abundant cation and the most common inorganic element in the human body. It is the principal component of the teeth and of bone. Functions of calcium are in relation to blood coagulation, neuromuscular excitability, cellular adhesiveness, transmission of nerve impulses, maintenance of cell membrane function, activation of enzymes, and hormone function, as well as skeletal integrity.[49]

Calcium Deficiency

Calcium deficiency in the elderly is commonly associated with osteomalacia and osteoporosis, and may be associated with hypocalcemia and tetany. However, neither hypocalcemia nor tetany are uniform signs of calcium deficiency since with mobilization of calcium from the skeleton, serum levels of calcium can be normal or elevated. Further, tetany may be due to magnesium deficiency.

Calcium depletion can be induced by drugs that exert their effects through one of the following mechanisms: (1) reduction in calcium absorption; (2) reduction in vitamin D absorption; (3) production of a phosphorus depletion syndrome; and (4) potentiation of renal excretion of calcium. Drugs used in the elderly that cause calcium malabsorption are those that cause intestinal mucosal damage. Neomycin, when administered orally in doses of 3–12 g/day for three to seven days, causes a reversible malabsorption syndrome with increased fecal excretion of calcium, as well as fat, nitrogen, sodium, potassium, and vitamin B_{12}.[50–52]

Primary calcium malabsorption may be due to neomycin, particularly when intake of neomycin is prolonged. It may be related to inhibition of pancreatic lipase, with subsequent development of steatorrhea and production of insoluble calcium soaps that are lost in the feces.[53] Malabsorption of calcium can also occur with administration of colchicine in doses that cause diarrhea and steatorrhea.[54]

Secondary drug-induced calcium malabsorption is due to drugs that decrease the absorption of vitamin D and also drugs that interfere with the conversion of vitamin D to the hepatic metabolite (25-hydroxycholecalciferol). It has long been known that when mineral oil is ingested in large amounts, it can cause a substantial reduction in the absorption of vitamin D, leading to the development of osteomalacia.[55,56]

There have been no recent reports of osteomalacia induced by mineral oil, which may indicate that excessive intake is no longer a problem or that osteomalacia due to this cause has been overlooked.

Long-term anticonvulsant therapy with phenytoin or phenobarbital has been shown to cause intestinal calcium malabsorption, with the development of osteomalacia. Wahl et al.[57] reported that fractional calcium absorption is low in patients receiving these anticonvulsant drugs even when the serum level of 25-hydroxycholecalciferol is within normal limits and when the response of bone and the kidney of parathyroid hormone is normal.

Osteomalacia has been reported in epileptics receiving phenytoin and phenobarbital with or without primidone.[58] Many investigators have attributed this drug-induced vitamin D deficiency to metabolism of vitamin D to more polar, inactive forms that are then excreted into the urine.[59,60] However, this hypothesis has not been proven.

Ray and Rao[61] reported a study of the calcium status of 36 elderly epileptic patients who were being treated with combined anticonvulsant drugs including phenytoin and phenobarbital three times daily for periods ranging from six weeks to ten years. In none of these 36 patients did hypocalcemia develop, and serum phosphorus levels also remained within normal limits, though alkaline phosphatase activity was slightly increased in 42% of the cases. It was concluded by the authors that hypocalcemia and osteomalacia are rare in elderly patients with seizure disorders who receive anticonvulsant therapy, either for short or prolonged periods.

Despite this report, it should be recognized that geriatric patients in long-term care facilities as well as housebound elderly are vulnerable or at risk for the development of osteomalacia due to the combined effects of low dietary intake of vitamin D if milk intake is low, lack of exposure to sunlight, and intake of anticonvulsants that cause calcium depletion either because of a primary effect of the drugs on calcium absorption, or due to secondary vitamin D deficiency, which is presently of uncertain etiology.[62,63]

Corticosteroid drugs also impair calcium absorption and also cause mobilization of calcium from the skeleton with resultant hypercalciuria. In steroid-induced osteopenia, there are several etiological components, among which are a reduced serum level of the renal metabolite of vitamin D, 1,25-dihydroxycholecalciferol.[64]

Diuretics, which are the commonest therapeutic drugs prescribed for the elderly, may cause calcium depletion and associated hypocalcemia. Furosemide and ethacrynic acid decrease serum calcium levels and cause hypercalciuria.[65] Furosemide has been administered intravenously to treat hypercalcemia, and the drug has caused a reduction in serum calcium in some patients, but complications of this treatment have included hypomagnesemia and a decline in renal function.[66]

An oral laxative containing phosphate, used to prepare patients for barium enemas, has been shown to elevate serum phosphorus levels, which is followed by a decrease in serum calcium levels.[67]

Case reports have also appeared in the literature in which middle-aged and elderly patients have developed hypocalcemia during laxative abuse. In such cases, it has been suggested that the hypocalcemia is secondary to calcium malabsorption associated with steatorrhea.[68]

Osteomalacia can also develop secondarily to antacid abuse when patients have taken excessive amounts of antacids containing aluminum and magnesium hydroxide. In these cases, insoluble aluminum and magnesium phosphates are formed by combination with dietary phosphate in the gastrointestinal tract. Antacid abuse leads primarily to phosphate depletion and secondarily to calcium depletion and the development of osteomalacia. However, both phosphate depletion and osteomalacia associated with excess intake of antacids appear to be somewhat uncommon if the small number of reports in the literature in any way reflect incidence.

Drugs causing calcium depletion, hypocalcemia, and bone mineral loss are shown in Table 6-3.

MAGNESIUM

Magnesium is required in all reactions requiring ATP (adenosine monophosphate). It is required for the conversion of ATP to cyclic AMP by adenylate cyclase. Magnesium is essential to normal neuromuscular function.[69]

Magnesium Deficiency

Magnesium deficiency is most often seen in elderly patients with diarrheal disorders leading to malabsorption and increased intestinal magnesium losses. Elderly alcoholics may also become magnesium deficient due to high renal losses

Table 6-3. Drugs Causing Calcium Depletion, Hypocalcemia, and Bone Mineral Loss

Calcium Depletion	Hypocalcemia	Bone Mineral Loss*
Neomycin	Furosemide	
Colchicine	Ethacrynic acid	Phenobarbital (OM)
	Phenolphthalein	Phenytoin (OM)
		Corticosteroids (OP)
		Aluminum and magnesium hydroxide (OM)

OM = osteomalacia
OP = osteoporosis

of magnesium. It is unlikely that an elderly person would become magnesium deficient because of a dietary deficiency of this mineral; as shown by Greger et al.,[70] certain foods commonly eaten by elderly people (including disabled elderly) because of low cost and no requirement for preparation are rich magnesium sources. Included among these foods are chocolate and breakfast cereals.

Intake of magnesium is likely to be inadequate in elderly patients who are unable or unwilling to eat, or in those who are receiving intravenous fluids that contain little or no magnesium. Clinical signs of magnesium deficiency include muscle weakness, tremors, depression, instability, and psychotic behavior. Seizures and tetany may occur.[71]

Drugs Causing Magnesium Depletion

Drugs that most often cause magnesium depletion in the elderly are digitalis and oral diuretics. Thiazide-induced hypomagnesemia occurs when the daily dose of the diuretic is high and when intake of dietary magnesium is low.[72] When elderly patients on diuretics are alcohol abusers, the risk of magnesium deficiency is higher because a high alcohol intake causes renal magnesium depletion.[73]

Hyperexcretion of magnesium developing during high and prolonged intake of the loop diuretics furosemide and ethacrynic acid is most likely to evoke magnesium deficiency in elderly patients with congestive heart failure who are anorectic. When hypomagnesemia occurs in elderly patients with congestive heart failure who are receiving digitalis as well as diuretics, digitalis toxicity with cardiac arrhythmia may be secondary to the magnesium deficiency. Tissue deficits of magnesium in patients on diuretic therapy for heart failure result from the combined effects of these drugs, digoxin intake, low dietary magnesium, and secondary aldosteronism.[74,75]

Severe magnesium deficiency is most likely to be the result of administration of nephrotoxic agents. Combined hypomagnesemia, hypokalemia, hypocalcemia, and alkalosis has developed in patients receiving gentamicin. Gentamicin-induced renal tubular damage has been exacerbated by cephalosporin antibiotics and by potassium deficiency. Additive or interactive effects of these risk factors for renal tubular injury also determine secondary magnesium deficiency.[76,77]

The cancer chemotherapeutic agent cisplatin (cis-platinum [II] dichlorodiamine) is also nephrotoxic and can cause magnesium deficiency. In cisplatin toxicity, there is both decreased glomerular filtration and loss of renal tubular absorptive capacity. The nephrotoxic effect of this drug and the associated magnesium deficiency are prevented by adequate hydration prior to and during the treatment period.[78,79]

Hypomagnesemia is associated with phosphate depletion and hypophosphatemia. Apparently the magnesium depletion is due to increased magnesium excretion in the urine secondary to the phosphate depletion, which, in the elderly, may occur with abuse of antacids containing aluminum hydroxide, because aluminum phosphate is formed in the intestine and is excreted in the feces.[71]

Drugs causing malabsorption with steatorrhea can also cause magnesium defi-

Table 6-4. Drugs Causing Magnesium Deficiency and Hypomagnesemia in the Elderly

Renal losses:	Thiazides
	Furosemide
	Ethacrynic acid
	Gentamicin
	Cisplatin
Gastrointestinal losses:	Neomycin
	Colchicine

ciency because of formation of magnesium soaps that are lost in the feces. Drugs taken by the elderly that can result in intestinal magnesium depletion include neomycin and colchicine.

Drugs causing magnesium deficiency and hypomagnesemia are shown in Table 6-4.

IRON

The major function of iron in the body is in the synthesis of hemoglobin and other hemes. Major causes of iron deficiency include low intake, malabsorption, and increased loss by bleeding. Drug-induced iron deficiency with development of iron deficiency anemia is commonly due to intake of drugs that cause gastrointestinal bleeding. Iron deficiency may be induced by chronic intake of aspirin or other non-narcotic analgesic drugs, such as indomethacin. These drugs cause erosions in the stomach and in the mucosa of the intestinal tract, from which there is continued blood loss. Chronic blood loss into the gastrointestinal tract, then, is the major cause of iron deficiency when these drugs are taken in high dosages, as is the case in elderly patients with arthritis.[80,81]

Aspirin also increases bleeding time. Mills et al.[82] have suggested that intestinal hemorrhage following ingestion of aspirin occurs because of the drug's antiplatelet effects leading to inhibition of platelet aggregation.[83]

ZINC

Zinc plays a critical role in the mechanism of action of many zinc metalloenzymes and also causes increase in the activity of nonmetallic enzymes. Zinc is essential to normal nucleic acid and protein metabolism and is also required for the stabilization of cell membranes.[84]

Zinc deficiency is due both to low intake, particularly in patients receiving parenteral nutrition, and to drugs. Zinc deficiency in the elderly occurs particularly in alcoholics. Alcoholics have a low intake of zinc and also excrete an excessive amount of zinc in their urine.

In the elderly, major signs of zinc deficiency include impaired healing of wounds and ulcers, including decubitus ulcers, scaly dermatitis of the face and limbs, and anorexia associated with loss of taste.[85]

Drugs such as penicillamine, which chelate metals such as zinc and copper, will induce depletion of zinc with long-term administration. Penicillamine is commonly administered for the management of rheumatoid arthritis, which may occur in the elderly quite frequently.[86]

Cardiac glycosides, such as digitalis, and also diuretics, particularly loop diuretics, can cause zinc depletion via the kidney. Whether or not severe zinc deficiency can be induced solely by intake of these drugs has, however, been disputed.[87]

DISCUSSON AND CONCLUSIONS

Drug groups and individual drugs that cause mineral depletion in the elderly are all in common use by geriatric patients living at home or in hospitals or extended care facilities. Several drugs that can lead to mineral deficiencies may be taken concurrently by patients on multiple-drug regimens. It is also significant that drugs used for different pharmacological purposes can have additive effects in producing mineral deficiencies. It is also notable that many of the symptoms and signs of mineral deficiencies mimic those that have traditionally been related to aging or to geriatric diseases.

Recognition of the risk of mineral deficiencies induced by drugs by physicians and other caregivers is essential. Present needs are also to develop improved screening methods for the recognition of mineral deficiencies in the elderly.

REFERENCES

1. Williamson J, Chopin JM: Adverse reactions to prescribed drugs in the elderly: A multicentre investigation. Age and Ageing 9:73–81, 1980.
2. Ouslander JG: Drug therapy in the elderly. Ann Intern Med 95:711–722, 1981.
3. Crooks J, Stevenson IH: Drug response in the elderly: Sensitivity and pharmacokinetic considerations. Age and Ageing 10:73–80, 1981.
4. Hansen JM, Kampmann J, Laursen H: Renal excretion of drugs in the elderly. Lancet 1:1170, 1970.
5. Cape RDT: Biological ageing. In Turner P (ed): Clinical Pharmacology and Therapeutics. Proceedings of the First World Conference on Clinical Pharmacology and Therapeutics, London, August, 1980. London, Macmillan, 1980, pp 89–97.
6. Holliday MA, Richardson KM, Portale A: Nutritional management of chronic renal disease. Med Clin N Am 63:945–962, 1979.
7. Warmold I, Lundholm K, Schirsten T: Energy balance and body composition in cancer patients. Cancer Res 38:1801–1807, 1978.
8. Flink EB: Mineral metabolism. In Kissin B, Begleiter H (eds).: The Biology of Alcoholism. Vol. 1, Biochemistry. New York: Plenum Press, 1971, pp 377–395.
9. Exton-Smith AN, Overstall PW: Geriatrics. Lancaster, England: MTP Press Ltd, 1979.
10. Nutrition and Health in Old Age: The Cross-Sectional Analysis of the Findings of a Survey Made in 1972/73 of Elderly People Who Had Been Studied in 1967/68. Department of Health and Social Security Publication No. 16. London, Her Majesty's Stationery Office, 1979.

11. Harper HA, Rodwell VW, Mayes PA: Water and mineral metabolism. In Review of Physiological Chemistry, 16th ed. Los Altos, Calif, Lange Medical Publications, 1977, pp 516–661.

12. Flear CTG, Gill GV, Burn J: Hyponatremia: Mechanisms and Management. Lancet 2:26–31, 1981.

13. Arieff AL, Llach F, Massry SG: Neurological manifestations and morbidity of hyponatremia: Correlation with rain water and electrolytes. Medicine 55:121–129, 1976.

14. Hantman D, Rossier B, Zohlman R, Schrier R: Rapid correction of hyponatremia in the syndrome of inappropriate secretion of antidiuretic hormone. An alternative treatment to hypertonic saline. Ann Intern Med 78:870–875, 1973.

15. Moses AM, Miller M: Drug-induced dilutional hyponatremia. New Engl J Med 291:1234–1239, 1974.

16. Hagen GA, Frawley TF: Hyponatremia due to sulfonylurea compounds. J Clin Endocrinol Metab 31:570–575, 1970.

17. Luethi A, Studer H: Antidiuretic action of chlorpropamide and tolbutamide. Minn Med 52:33–36, 1969.

18. Weissman PN, Schenkman L, Gregerman RI: Chlorpropamide hyponatremia: Drug-induced inappropriate antidiuretic-hormone activity. New Engl J Med 284:65–71, 1971.

19. Oldham RK, Pomeroy TC: Vincristine-induced syndrome of inappropriate secretion of antidiuretic hormones. South Med J 65:1010–1012, 1972.

20. Steele TH, Serpick AA, Block JB: Antidiuretic response to cyclophosphamide in man. J Pharmacol Exp Ther 185:245–253, 1973.

21. Rado JP: Water intoxication during carbamazepine treatment. Br Med J 3:479, 1973.

22. Luzecky MH, Burman KD, Schultz ER: The syndrome of inappropriate secretion of antidiuretic hormone associated with amitryptyline administration. South Med J 67: 495–497, 1974.

23. Ashraf N, Locksley R, Arieff AI: Thiazide-induced hyponatremia associated with death or neurological damage in outpatients. Am J Med 70:1163–1168, 1981.

24. Nicholls MG, Espinar EA, Hughes H, Rogers T: Effect of potassium-sparing diuretics on the renin-angiotensin-aldosterone system and potassium retention in heart failure. Br Heart J 38:1025–1030, 1976.

25. Nicholls MG, Espinar EA, Ikram H, Maslowski AH: Hyponatremia in congestive heart failure during treatment with Captopril. Br Med J 281:909, 1980.

26. Flear CTG, Singh CM: Hyponatremia and sick cells. Br J Anaesth 45:976–994, 1973.

27. Flear CTG, Bhattacharya SS, Singh CM: Solute and water exchange between cells and extracellular fluids in health and disturbances after trauma. J Parent Ent Nutr 4:98–120, 1980.

28. Thomas TH, Morgan DB, Swaminathan R: Severe hyponatremia: A study of 17 patients. Lancet 1:621–624, 1978.

29. Comis RJ, Miller M, Ginsberg SJ: Abnormalities in water homeostasis in small cell-anaplastic lung cancer. Cancer 45:2414–2421, 1980.

30. Trump DL: Serious hyponatremia in patients with cancer: Management with demeclocycline. Cancer 47:2908–2912, 1981.

31. Nardone DA, McDonald WJ, Girard DE: Mechanism of hypokalemia: Clinical correlation. Medicine 57:435–446, 1978.

32. Steen B. Hypokalemia, clinical spectrum and etiology. Acta Med Scand, suppl 647, pp 61–66, 1981.

33. Hollifield JW, Slaton PE: Thiazide diuretics, hypokalemia and cardiac arrhythmias. Acta Med Scand, suppl 647, pp 67–74, 1981.

34. Hamdy RC, Tovey J, Perera N: Hypokalemia and diuretics. Br Med J 1:1187, 1980.

35. Ramsey LE, Bayle P, Ramsay MH: Factors influencing serum potassium in treated hypertension. Quart J Med 46:401–410, 1977.
36. Fleming, BJ, Genuth SM, Gould AB, Kamionkowski MD: Laxative-induced hypokalemia, sodium depletion, and hyperreninemia. Ann Intern Med 83:60–62, 1975.
37. Levine D, Goode AW, Wingate DL: Purgative abuse associated with reversible cachexia, hypogammaglobulinemia, and finger clubbing. Lancet 1:919–920, 1981.
38. Thorn GW: Clinical considerations in the use of corticosteroids. New Engl J Med 274:775–781, 1966.
39. Srivastava LS, Werk EE, Thrasher K, et al.: Plasma cortisone concentration as measured by radioimmunoassay. J Clin Endocrinol Metab 36:937–943, 1973.
40. Smith MJH, Smith PK (eds): The Salicylates: A Critical Bibliographical Review. New York, Interscience, 1966.
41. Mazze RI, Cousins MJ: Combined nephrotoxicity of gentamicin and methoxyflurane anaesthesia: A case report. Br J Anaesth 45:394–398, 1973.
42. Drutz DJ, Tai TY, Cheng T, Hsieh WC: Hypokalemic rhabdomyolysis and myoglobinuria following amphotericin B therapy. JAMA 211:824–826, 1970.
43. O'Brien IAD, Fitzgerald-Fraser J, Lewin IG, Carrall AJM: Hypokalemia due to solbutamol overdosage. Br Med J 282:1515–1516, 1981.
44. Gungdogdu AS, Brown PM, Juul S, et al.: Comparison of the hormonal and metabolic effects of solbutamol infusion in normal subjects and in insulin-requiring diabetics. Lancet 2:1317–1321, 1979.
45. Granerus A-K, Jagenburg R, Svanborg A: Kaliuretic effects of L-dopa treatment in parkinsonian patients. Acta Med Scand 201:291–297, 1977.
46. Steiness E: Diuretics, digitalis and arrhythmias. Acta Med Scand, suppl 647, pp 75–85, 1981.
47. Katz FH, Eckert RC, Gebott MD: Hypokalemia caused by surreptitious self-administration of diuretics. Ann Intern Med 76:85–90, 1972.
48. Wrong O, Richards P: Psychiatric disturbance and electrolyte depletion. Lancet 1:421–422, 1968.
49. Avioli LW: Calcium and phosphorus. In Goodhart RS, Shills ME (eds): Modern Nutrition in Health and Disease, 6th ed. Philadelphia: Lea & Febiger, 1980, p 294.
50. Faloon WW, Chodos RB: Vitamin B_{12} absorption studies using colchicine, neomycin and continuous 57Co-B_{12} administration. Gastroenterology 56:1, 251, 1969.
51. Faloon WW: Effect of neomycin and kanamycin upon intestinal absorption. Ann NY Acad Sci 132:879–887, 1966.
52. Faloon WW: Drug production of intestinal malabsorption. NY State J Med 70:2189–2192, 1970.
53. Mehta SK, Wesser E, Sleisenger MA: The in vitro effect of bacterial metabolites and antibiotics on pancreatic lipase activity. Abs J Clin Invest 43:1252, 1964.
54. Race TR, Paes IC, Faloon WW: Intestinal malabsorption induced by oral colchicine: Comparison with neomycin and cathartic agents. Am J Med Sci 259:32–41, 1970.
55. Meulengracht E: Osteomalacia of the spinal column from deficient diet or from disease of the digestive tract. 3. Osteomalacia e abuse laxantium. Acta Med Scand 101:187–210, 1979.
56. Morgan JW: The harmful effects of mineral oil (liquid petrolatum) purgatives. JAMA 117:1335–1336, 1941.
57. Wahl TO, Gobuty AH, Lukert BP: Long-term anticonvulsant therapy and intestinal calcium absorption. Clin Pharmacol Ther 30:506–512, 1981.
58. Dent CE, Richens A, Rowe DJF, Stamp TCB: Osteomalacia with long-term anticonvul-

sant therapy in epilepsy. Br Med J 4:69–72, 1970.

59. Hahn TJ, Birge SJ, Sharp CR, Avioli LV: Phenobarbital-induced alterations in vitamin D metabolism. J Clin Invest 51:741–748, 1972.

60. Hahn TJ, Hendin BA, Scharp CR, Haddad JG Jr: Effect of chronic anticonvulsant therapy on serum 25-hydroxycalciferol levels in adults. New Engl J Med 287:900–909, 1972.

61. Ray AK, Rao DB: Calcium metabolism in elderly epileptic patients during anticonvulsant therapy. J Am Geriat Soc 22:222–225, 1974.

62. Corless D, Boucher BJ, Beer M, et al.: Vitamin D status in long-stage geriatric patients. Lancet 1:1404–1406, 1975.

63. Roe DA: Drug-Induced Nutritional Deficiencies. Westport, Conn, AVI Publishing, 1976, pp 211–221.

64. Chesney RW, Mazees RB, Hamstra AJ, et al.: Reduction of serum-1,15-dihydroxy-vitamin-D in children receiving glucocorticoids. Lancet 2:1123–1125, 1978.

65. Eknoyan G, Suki WN, Martinez-Maldonardo M: Effect of diuretics on urinary excretion of phosphate, calcium and magnesium in thyroparathyroidectomized dogs. J Lab Clin Med 76:25, 1970.

66. Suki WN, Yium JJ, Von Minden M, et al.: Acute treatment of hypercalcemia with furosemide. New Engl J Med 283:836–840, 1970.

67. Wiberg JJ, Turner GG, Nuttall FQ: Effect of phosphate or magnesium cathartics on serum calcium: Observations in normal calcemic patients. Arch Intern Med 138:1114–1116, 1978.

68. Frame B, Guiang HL, Frost HM, Reynolds WA: Osteomalacia induced by laxative (phenolphthalein) ingestion. Arch Intern Med 128:794–796, 1971.

69. Shils ME: Magnesium. In Goodhart RS, Shils ME (eds): Modern Nutrition in Health and Disease, 6th ed. Philadelphia: Lea & Febiger, 1980, pp 310–313.

70. Greger JL, Marhefka S, Geissler AH: A research note: Magnesium content of selected foods. J Food Sci 43:1610–1612, 1978.

71. Rude RK, Singer FR: Magnesium deficiency and excess. Ann Rev Med 32:245–259, 1981.

72. Duarte CG: Effects of chlorothiazide and amipramizide (MK 870) on the renal excretion of calcium phosphate and magnesium. Metabolism 17:420–429, 1968.

73. Sullivan JF, Lankford HG, Swartz MJ, Farrell C: Magnesium metabolism in alcoholism. Am J Clin Nutr 13:297–303, 1963.

74. Lim P, Jacob E: Magnesium deficiency in patients on long-term diuretic therapy for heart failure. Br Med J 2:620–622, 1972.

75. Wacker WEC, Parisi AF: Magnesium metabolism. New Engl J Med 278:712–721, 771–776, 1968.

76. Bar RS, Wilson HE, Mazzaferri EL: Hypomagnesemic hypocalcemia secondary to renal magnesium wasting: A possible consequence of high-dose gentamicin therapy. Ann Intern Med 82:646–649, 1975.

77. Luft FC, Patel V, Yum M, Kleit SA: Antimicrobial agents. Chemotherapy 9:831–839, 1976.

78. Schilsky R, Anderson T: Hypomagnesemia secondary to cisdiammine-chloroplatinum II administration. Ann Intern Med 90:929–931, 1979.

79. Stark JJ, Howell SB: Nephrotoxicity of cisplatinum (II) dichlorodiammine. Clin Pharmacol Ther 23:461–466, 1978.

80. Leonards JR, Levy G: Gastrointestinal blood loss during prolonged aspirin administration. New Engl J Med 289:1020–1022, 1973.

81. Bordman PL, Hart ED: Side effects of indomethacin. Ann Rheum Dis 26:127–132, 1967.
82. Mills DG, Borda IT, Philip RB, Eldridge G: Effect of in vitro aspirin on blood platelets of gastrointestinal bleeders. Clin Pharmacol Ther 15:167–192, 1974.
83. Watson Buchanan W, Rooney PJ, Rennie AN: Aspirin and the salicylates. Clin Rheumat Dis 5:499–539, 1979.
84. Li T-K, Vallee BL: The biochemical and nutritional roles of other trace elements. In Goodhart RS, Shills ME (eds): Modern Nutrition in Health and Disease, 6th ed. Philadelphia: Lea & Febiger, 1980, pp 419–428.
85. Jacob RA: Zinc and copper. Clinics in Lab Med 1:743–756, 1981.
86. Day AT, Golding JR, Lee PN, Butterworth AD: Penicillamine in rheumatoid disease: A long-term study. Br Med J 1:180–183, 1974.
87. Wester P.O: Zinc during diuretic treatment. Lancet 1:578, 1975.

7 | Adverse Nutritional Effects of OTC Drug Use in the Elderly

Daphne A. Roe

The elderly are frequent users and misusers both of prescription and of non-prescription drugs. Chien et al.[1] found that in a sample of 244 individuals over 60 years of age, the most commonly used drugs were analgesics (66.6%), cardiovascular drugs (33.5%), laxatives (30.6%), vitamins (29.3%), antacids (26.4%), and antianxiety agents (22.3%). In this study, 83% of the sample were taking two or more drugs, and over-the-counter (OTC) drugs accounted for 40% of the total medications used.

Guttman,[2] in a similar study of 441 elderly people, found that the most frequently used classes of medications were cardiovascular drugs (61.3%), sedatives and tranquilizers (16.6%), antiarthritic preparations (12.1%), and gastrointestinal medications (11.4%). Over-the-counter drugs were taken by 61% of these people, of whom 31.7% were taking analgesics and 7.1%, laxatives.

Several classes of OTC drugs may induce adverse nutritional effects. Among such drug groups, those most commonly reviewed in the literature are antacids, laxatives, and analgesics. Indeed, on the basis of an assortment of good and bad evidence, it has been strongly suggested that drug-induced malnutrition in the elderly is most commonly due to their excessive use of these OTC drugs. It should, however, be pointed out that not all studies suggesting that excessive use of either antacids, laxatives, or non-narcotic analgesics could lead to malnutrition have actually separated out other factors that could impair nutritional status, including an inadequate diet and the effects of physical disease, as well as the role of prescription drugs having adverse nutritional effects.

This chapter makes a critical review of the more recent literature describing the role of OTC drug use in the development of malnutrition. In order to set the scene for such a review, it is necessary to discuss reasons for OTC drug use and misuse by the elderly, and also to specify which drug or drug combinations are frequently taken.

ANTACIDS

Antacids in common use are those that are mixtures of aluminum and magnesium hydroxide, with or without magnesium carbonate, and others in which the chief acid ingredient is sodium bicarbonate. In the *Physicians' Desk Reference for Nonprescription Drugs,*[3] the actions of several of these antacids are described by such phrases as "relieves and soothes acid indigestion, heartburn, and sour stomach," under the heading "Interactions." In this reference, it is emphasized that antacids should not be taken concurrently with tetracycline. However, there is no other mention of drug/nutrient interactions. For each antacid preparation, under the heading "Doses and Administration, a Guideline," is given when the tablets or liquid should be taken and how large the total dosage should be within a 24-hour period. Antacids that contain defoamers are stated to relieve "gas."

Elderly people taking antacids may do so under physician's orders. Medical reasons for taking antacids on a regular basis and at defined intervals include end-stage renal disease, for which antacids are given in order to control hyperphosphatemia, and peptic ulcer. In the treatment of peptic ulcer, the goal of antacid therapy is to "modify" gastric acidity to yield a gastric pH of 3.5, at which point the activity of pepsin is lost. It has been pointed out by McHardy[4] that any claims that antacids "coat" the lining of the stomach and exert a beneficial effect because of this "coating" are unfounded.

There are many antacids on the market. Almost any of these preparations can give effective relief from peptic ulcer pain.[5] Fordtran[6] presented evidence that the usual cause of failure of antacids in this regard has been insufficient dosage.

In the past, it has been generally accepted by gastroenterologists, that in order to use antacids effectively in the management of active peptic ulcer disease, it is necessary that the patient take the antacid one hour and three hours postprandially and also at bedtime. Certain authors have also advocated a "wake-up dose" during the night. Actual amounts of an antacid preparation to be taken clearly must vary with the preparation, but with the common liquid antacids containing aluminum and magnesium hydroxide, it is usually suggested that individual dosages should be between 45 and 60 ml.[4]

In considering whether these dosages of antacids pose a nutritional risk, it is important to note that Roth and Berger[7] showed very convincingly that more than 50% of peptic ulcer patients do not comply with antacid schedules, even when under hospital conditions.

Antacid Use in the Elderly

Although high doses of antacid mixtures are not infrequently prescribed in the elderly to combat hyperphosphatemia occurring as a complication of end-stage renal disease, much more commonly, elderly men and women will take antacids without specific medical advice in order to relieve symptoms that are variably described as indigestion, flatulence, heart problems, gas, bloating, and gastric discomfort. Antacids may be taken by older people whenever unpleasant symptoms occur after eating, regardless of the cause. Underlying causes of these symptoms may be related to the gastrointestinal tract, including hiatus hernia, esophageal or peptic ulcers, systemic sclerosis involving the esophagus, and alcoholic gastritis. Antacids may also be taken for relief of epigastric discomfort related to angina and congestive heart failure, or dyspnea related to emphysema.

Adverse Metabolic and Nutritional Effects of Antacid Use

The Milk-Alkali Syndrome   The milk-alkali syndrome occurs as a complication of excessive ingestion of soluble alkali and milk. It is characterized by hypercalcemia without hypercalciuria or hyperphosphaturia. Renal insufficiency with azotemia may develop with alkalosis. Symptoms include anorexia, nausea, vomiting, headache, and weakness. Signs include band keratitis due to deposition of calcium in the cornea. The milk-alkali syndrome has been reported in patients taking large amounts of sodium bicarbonate or calcium carbonate. Elderly patients are at risk, particularly those who have preexistent renal insufficiency.[8,9]

Hypophosphatemia   Hypophosphatemia has been reported with excessive use of antacids containing aluminum and magnesium hydroxide.[10] Phosphate depletion associated with excess intake of antacids would appear to be uncommon if a number of reports actually reflect incidence.[11] However, it seems very possible that antacid-induced hypophosphatemia is often unrecognized because of insidious development of weakness, which is a sign of metabolic disorder. This may be ascribed to other age-related causes in the elderly.

Aluminum and magnesium hydroxides form nonabsorbable phosphates in the gut lumen. Secondary osteomalacia may develop,[12] causing bone pain and/or difficulty in walking, which, again, are easy to misdiagnose in the elderly.[11] Hypomagnesemia leading to tetany may be secondary to phosphate depletion.[13]

Sodium Overload   Sodium overload, with development of congestive heart failure, can result from intake of antacids containing sodium bicarbonate. The risk is greatest in elderly patients with preexisting heart disease who also consume high-sodium diets. Other etiological factors include intake of drinking water that is high in sodium because of contamination, usually from water softeners, and intake of other high-sodium drugs and such drugs as the antihypertensive agent diazoxide, which increases the proximal tubular reabsorption of sodium.[14,15]

Magnesium Overload   Magnesium intoxication has been reported in patients with chronic renal failure who have been taking magnesium-containing antacids.[16,17] Signs of magnesium intoxication include nausea, vomiting and flushing, impaired respiratory function, and partial or complete heart block. Lithium carbonate, used in the management of manic-depressive psychosis, may induce hypermagnesemia.[18]

Aluminum Toxicity   There has been some speculation as to whether aluminum-containing antacids can cause aluminum toxicity. In normal people, whether young or elderly, aluminum is virtually excluded from absorption from the skin, the lungs, or the gastrointestinal tract.[19] However, in patients with renal failure, absorption of small amounts of aluminum may cause dialysis dementia. Dialysis dementia is a progressive, usually fatal organic brain syndrome that has been reported in patients with end-stage renal disease who are undergoing repeated hemodialysis. It is considered that the syndrome is multifactorial, occurring as a consequence of aluminum loading, renal failure, and abnormalities in the blood/brain barrier. Concentrations of aluminum in the cerebral cortex are elevated. Aluminum loading may be due to entrance of aluminum salts into the body via the water used in the dialysis procedure or to administration of aluminum hydroxide. Arieff et al.[20] showed that in renal patients and in laboratory animals (dogs), aluminum levels in the brain can be elevated by renal failure as well as by aluminum hydroxide loading.

Whereas aluminum can be absorbed from the gastrointestinal tract after administration of aluminum-containing antacids, retention is greater in renal patients than in normal individuals.[21]

Folate Malabsorption   In a 1971 study by Benn et al.[22] in which jejunal pH was measured, findings were that when the pH of the jejunum was rendered more alkaline by administration of sodium bicarbonate, folic acid absorption was decreased. The authors, however, did not carry out direct measurements of folic acid absorption, but defined the rise in plasma folate after a given dose as an indirect measure of folic acid absorption.

When a similar type of investigation was performed by Perry and Chanarin,[23] no evidence was obtained that sodium bicarbonate interfered with folate absorption when the vitamin was administered in the monoglutamate form. Indeed, serum folate levels were higher after a folate dose (15 mg) when bicarbonate (10 g) was administered.

Later, however, MacKenzie and Russell,[24] using a triple-lumen technique, were able to demonstrate that when the jejunal pH was rendered more alkaline, folic acid was less well absorbed both in normal subjects and in patients with celiac disease.

Halsted,[25] after reviewing animal and human studies of effects of intestinal pH on folate absorption, commented that since folate absorption is enhanced when it is in a nonpolar form (between pH 6.0 and 6.5), any change in pH outside this range, whether acidic or alkaline directed, would decrease folate absorption.

Blair et al.[26] investigated effects of change in surface pH on folate absorption, using rat everted gut sacs. They found that when proximal intestinal mucosal pH was plotted against folate transport, a significant association could be demonstrated even though the relationship did not fit a simple linear regression model.

Although, in at least some of the studies cited, information was obtained that alkalinization of the proximal small intestine depresses folate absorption under test conditions, no clinical studies have been carried out to evaluate effects of antacid usage on folate absorption or folate status. The possibility exists, however, that in elderly people who have decreased gastric acid production and also take antacids, such as sodium bicarbonate, folate absorption might be reduced.

LAXATIVES

Laxatives and cathartics have been provisionally classified by Fingl and Preston[27] into five groups: (1) agents that alter electrolyte transport; (2) agents that alter intestinal motility; (3) agents that alter electrolyte transport and motility; (4) osmotic agents; and (5) bulk-forming agents. However, as these authors admit, this grouping overlooks the fact that in the present state of knowledge, misclassification is possible because the mechanism of action has not been identified using an appropriate methodology. Further, it is suggested that a more satisfactory means to describe the pharmacological action of laxatives would be at the cellular level and in relation to effects on gastrointestinal hormones.

Castor oil and dioctyl sodium sulfosuccinate have been considered together because of surfactant effects. Ricinoleic acid, the active metabolite of castor oil, as well as other anionic surface active agents, inhibit the absorption of sodium and glucose and convert sodium and water absorption into net secretion. These compounds stimulate adenylate cyclase, inhibit sodium potassium adenosine triphosphatase, and increase membrane permeability.[28] Dioctyl sulfosuccinate has surfactant properties that are similar to those of castor oil and bile acids. Additionally, it may increase the hydration of the feces.[29] The anthroquinone drugs, such as senna and cascara, and diphenylmethane derivatives, such as phenolphthalein, are common laxatives used extensively by the elderly. These drugs affect both electrolyte transport and intestinal motility. They reduce sodium absorption and convert net sodium and water absorption into secretion. Evidence suggests that they also affect intestinal mucosal permeability. They exert their effects at lower concentrations on the colon than on the small intestine.[30]

Saline cathartics include magnesium and sodium sulfate. These have commonly been regarded as osmotic laxatives, which act by drawing water into the colon. More recently it has been suggested that the saline laxatives function in part by virtue of the fact that they induced release of cholecystokinin in the duodenum. The net effects include increased pancreatic secretion as well as increase in secretion and motility of the small intestine.[31,32]

Mineral oil is a mixture of liquid hydrocarbons obtained from petroleum. The oil is indigestible and largely nonadsorbable from the intestine. Mineral oil functions as a stool softener and also has laxative properties in that it may inhibit or reduce water reabsorption from the colon.[33]

Natural and semisynthetic polysaccharides and cellulose have been used as bulking agents. Bulk-forming agents commonly used include bran, methylcellulose, ispaghula, as well as psyllium seeds. Bulk-forming agents increase stool bulk, as the name suggests, and may decrease intestinal transit time. It has further been claimed that they decrease intraluminal pressure and relieve symptoms related to constipation or to irritable bowel syndrome.[34]

In a study comparing effects of bran and ispaghula in constipated elderly patients,[35] both the ispaghula and the bran increased the wet and dry stool weight. There were no serious side effects and no change in colonic pressures. The authors presented evidence that these bulking agents have therapeutic advanges over regular laxatives for use in elderly constipated patients.

Laxative Use in the Elderly

Laxative use increases with age. Reasons for laxative use are[36]

1. Simple constipation due to a low-fiber diet
2. Chronic cardiac or respiratory disease in which physical distress, including dyspnea and/or pain, occurs with attempts to expel hard fecal masses
3. Diseases of the colon and rectum, including irritable bowel syndrome, cancer of the colon or rectum associated with partial obstruction, and hemorrhoids
4. Long-term use and abuse of laxatives
5. Intake of drugs that are constipating
6. Bowel obsessions

Adverse Nutritional Effects of Laxatives

Hypokalemia and Potassium Deficiency Hypokalemia is associated with laxative abuse because of loss of potassium into the gastrointestinal tract and failure of potassium reabsorption from the colon. Elderly patients ingesting excessive amounts of phenolphthalein, bisacodyl, and senna have been reported with severe hypokalemia for which the cause was undiscovered until their habit of laxative abuse was suspected and/or proved.[37,38] In elderly patients, the risks of hypokalemia and potassium deficiency, with the attendant hazards of cardiac arrhythmias, digitalis toxicity, and hyperglycemia, are associated with concurrent use of laxatives and thiazide or loop diuretics.[14]

Malabsorption Syndromes Malabsorption syndromes have been reported in laxative abusers, particularly in those who take excessive amounts of phenolphthalein or bisacodyl. Frame et al.[39] described a woman whose massive and prolonged intake of phenolphthalein resulted in osteomalacia. In this case, impaired absorption of xylose suggested the malabsorption state. Discontinuation of the phenylphthalein relieved the signs and symptoms of her vitamin D deficiency. It has been suggested by Heizer et al.[40] that the malabsorption may be related to loss of structural integrity of the intestinal epithelial cells secondary to potassium depletion.

Whereas such a loss of structural integrity provides an attractive explanation of the protein-losing enteropathy that may occur coincidentally with malabsorption in laxative abusers, this mechanism has not been demonstrated experimentally.[41]

Malabsorption of fat-soluble vitamins and beta carotene has long been known to occur with excessive intake of mineral oil, and studies have indicated that mineral oil impairs absorption, particularly of vitamins A, D, and K.[42-45] Curtis and Ballmer[46] studied human volunteers and showed that when beta carotene was taken concurrently with mineral oil, it was dissolved in the oil and not absorbed. Osteomalacia from excessive mineral oil intake has been documented.[47]

NON-NARCOTIC ANALGESICS

Aspirin

Aspirin and salicylate mixtures containing aspirin have long been known to produce gastrointestinal side effects. Estimates of the incidence of gastrointestinal side effects vary from about 5% to 6%[48] to more than 30%.[49] Varied incidence of side effects is undoubtedly due to differences in dose and dosage schedules.

Use of Aspirin by the Elderly Indications for use of aspirin by the elderly are several. Most commonly, aspirin is used to relieve pain, particularly pain associated with arthritis and other musculoskeletal disorders. Common use of aspirin in these disorders is related to the generally excellent analgesic and anti-inflammatory properties of the drug in younger people. However, the anti-inflammatory effects of aspirin in chronic joint disease of the elderly are not outstanding even when doses as high as 3 g/day are ingested.[50] The anti-inflammatory effects of aspirin are related to the inhibitory effects of the drug on prostaglandin synthesis.[51]

Elderly people may take aspirin on medical advice as a preventive of recurrent myocardial infarcts or to avert transient ischemic cerebral episodes. These therapeutic uses of aspirin are justified in that the drug has an antiplatelet effect and may prevent or admonish the risk of venous or thrombus formation.[52,53]

Nonspecific use of aspirin is common among elderly as well as younger people. Aspirin is widely taken for relief of such symptoms as headache, insomnia, nervousness, hangover, cold, cough, sore throat, and pain or discomfort unrelated to musculoskeletal disease.

Adverse Nutritional Effects of Aspirin It has long been known that aspirin may cause iron deficiency anemia by inducing blood loss from the GI tract. Blood loss is explained in part by erosions in the gastrointestinal mucosa causing capillary hemorrhage, and also by prolongation of bleeding time, which occurs with aspirin intake in certain individuals.[54,55]

Whereas it is accepted that iron deficiency anemia is a rather common adverse outcome of heavy aspirin usage, particularly in the elderly, there is also evidence that megaloblastic anemia due to folate deficiency may possibly occur with heavy aspirin use. Folic acid deficiency has been demonstrated in patients with rheumatoid arthritis, who commonly received therapeutic doses of aspirin.[56]

Alter et al.[57] reported decreased serum folate levels in 71% of 51 patients with rheumatoid arthritis. Eleven of these patients were studied further, and it was

Table 7-1. Etiological Factors and Outcomes Related to Primary Metabolic/Nutritional Effects of Antacid Use and Abuse

Etiological Factors and Outcomes	Metabolic and Nutritional Effects					
	Milk-Alkali Syndrome	Phosphate Depletion	Sodium Overload	Magnesium Overload	Aluminum Toxicity	Folate Malabsorption
Antacid	Na bicarb	Al/Mg	Na bicarb	Mg hydrox	Al hydrox	Na bicarb
Dose in relation to food	High dose with milk	With food	Not related	Not related	Not related	With food folate
Other drugs				Lithium carbonate		Alcohol
Disease present	Renal failure	Renal failure	Heart disease	Renal failure	Renal failure	IBD
Procedures				Dialysis	Dialysis	
Dietary characteristics	Milk diet		High sodium			Folate deficient
Adverse outcomes	Renal failure	Osteomalacia	Congestive heart failure	Heart block	Dementia	Megaloblastic anemia

shown that they had an abnormally rapid plasma clearance of tritium-labeled folic acid. These patients were all taking aspirin. There were other rheumatoid arthritis patients not taking aspirin who had normal folate binding and clearance.

Acetaminophen

Acetaminophen is a non-narcotic analgesic that may be used as an aspirin substitute. Abuse of this drug can result in an analgesic nephropathy that can result in chronic azotemia. The renal lesion consists in an interstitial nephritis with papillary necrosis. Patients with this disorder are "salt losers"; that is, they are unable to conserve body sodium. The risk of severe sodium depletion is increased when there is an intercurrent gastrointestinal disorder characterized by further sodium and water loss.[58] Severe hyponatremia in the elderly may be from combined effects of acetaminophen and acute gastroenteritis.

GENERAL DISCUSSION AND CONCLUSIONS

The hypothesis that malnutrition in the elderly is commonly due to drugs is based on knowledge of this group's excessive use of OTC and prescription drugs, including laxatives, antacids, and non-narcotic analgesics. There is information that these drugs can cause vitamin and mineral depletion.[41] This review has focused on adverse nutritional outcomes of OTC drug misuse; perhaps insufficient emphasis has been placed on the multifactorial etiology of these forms of drug-induced malnutrition. Risks of malnutrition in elderly people taking excessive amounts of OTC drugs, such as antacids, laxatives, and non-narcotic analgesics, are greatest in marginal malnutrition if dietary origin is present. Timing of drugs in relation to meals may also be an important determinant of nutritional depletion.

Table 7-2. Etiological Factors and Outcomes Related to Adverse Nutritional Effects of Laxative Use

Etiological Factors and Outcomes	Hypokalemia and Potassium Deficiency	Malabsorption Syndromes	Protein-Losing Enteropathy
Laxative	Phenolphthalein Bisacodyl Senna	Phenolphthalein Bisacodyl Senna Mineral oil	Phenolphthalein
Dose and dose frequency	High dose	High dose	High dose
Other drugs	Diuretics	Laxative taken with or after food	
Disease present	---------------- Depression or paranoid psychosis -----------------		
Dietary characteristics	Low potassium		Low protein
Adverse outcomes	Digitalis toxicity Arrythmias	Osteomalacia	Protein malnutrition

Table 7-3. Factors Contributing to Vitamin and Mineral Depletion in Elderly Individuals Receiving Non-narcotic Analgesics

Etiological Factors	Iron Deficiency	Nutritional Impairment Folate Depletion	Sodium Depletion
Drug	Aspirin	Aspirin	Acetaminophen
Disease	Rheumatoid arthritis; IBD; Ca colon; other GI diseases blood loss	Rheumatoid arthritis; IBD; malabsorption syndromes	Gastroenteritis
Diet	Low calorie, low iron	Low folate	Sodium restriction

Phosphate depletion associated with antacids occurs when the antacid is taken in close proximity to mealtimes. Usage of other drugs is also important. For example, potassium depletion is more likely to be an outcome of laxative use in patients who are also taking diuretics. Excessive alcohol intake may also influence the risk of nutritional deficiency. Folate deficiency, which is common in alcoholics, may be worsened when there is heavy intake of sodium bicarbonate–containing antacids that impair folate absorption.[59]

Tables 7-1–7-3 summarize risk factors for adverse nutritional side effects of antacids, laxatives, and OTC analgesics.

Although it is true that certain elderly people may take excessive amounts of antacids or laxatives, or even non-narotic analgesics because of obsessional ideas about need to prevent gastric distress, constipation, or headache, other elderly may take these drugs because they need symptomatic relief. Drug education and avoidance of misuse of OTC drugs is necessary and, hopefully, feasible. When OTC drugs are taken with justification, then it is necessary that they be timed appropriately with relation to mealtimes. Martin and Mead[60] found that color-coded bottles or pill boxes (colors indicating times for drugs to be taken) have a significant effect in reducing timing misuse of drugs.

We have recently proposed that drug education of the elderly with relation to OTC medications could appropriately be carried out using videotape or television. Aims of such a program would be to inform elderly people about the health risks of the misuse of OTC drugs, to explain why such drugs should not be taken with food or nutrient supplements, and to impress the elderly with the need to check *all* medications in use, including OTC drugs, with a local pharmacist.

REFERENCES

1. Chien CP, Townsend EJ, Townsend A: Substance use and abuse among the community elderly: The medical aspect. Addict Dis 3:357–372, 1978.
2. Guttman P: Patterns of legal drug use by older Americans. Addict Dis 3:337–356, 1978.
3. *Physicians' Desk Reference for Nonprescription Drugs,* 1st ed. Oradell, NJ, Cole Economics Co, 1980.

4. McHardy G: Medical management of uncomplicated duodenal ulcer: Current views and newer drugs. In Berk JE (ed): Developments in Digestive Diseases; Clinical Evidence. Philadelphia: Lea & Febiger, 1977, pp 47–57.

5. The Medical Letter. Vol. 13, no. 13, November 12, 1971.

6. Fordtran JS: Acid rebound. New Engl J Med 279:900, 1968.

7. Roth HP, Berger BG: Studies on patient cooperation in ulcer treatment. 1. Observation of acute as compared to prescribed antacid intake on a hospital ward. Gastroenterology 38:631–633, 1960.

8. Kirsner JB: Acid-peptic disease: Peptic ulcer. In Beeson PB, McDermott W (eds): Cecil-Loeb's Textbook of Medicine, 11th ed. Philadelphia and London: W B Saunders, 1963, pp 906–907.

9. Randall RE Jr, Strauss MB, McNeeley WF: The milk-alkali syndrome. Arch Intern Med 107:163–181, 1961.

10. Lotz M, Zisman E, Bartter C: Evidence for a phosphorus-depletion syndrome in man. New Engl J Med 278:409–415, 1968.

11. Parfitt AM, Gallagher JC, Heaney RP, et al.: Vitamin D and bone health in the elderly. Amer J Clin Nutr 36:1014–1031, 1982.

12. Insogna KL, Bordley DR, Caro JF, Lockwood DH: Osteomalacia and weakness from excessive antacid. JAMA 244:2544–2546, 1980.

13. Rude RK, Singer FR: Magnesium deficiency and excess. Ann Rev Med 32:245–259, 1981.

14. Roe DA: Drug interference with the assessment of nutritional status. Clin Lab Med 1:647–664, 1981.

15. Bartorelli C, Gargano N, Leonnetti G, Zanchetti A: Hypotensive and renal effects of diazoxide: A sodium-retaining benzothiadiazine compound. Circulation 27:895–903, 1963.

16. Hirschfelder AD: Clinical manifestations of high and low plasma magnesium. JAMA 102:1138–1141, 1934.

17. Wacker WEC, Parisi AF: Magnesium metabolism. New Engl J Med 278:658–663, 712–717, 771–776, 1968.

18. Nielson J: Magnesium-lithium studies: Serum and erythrocyte magnesium in patients with manic states. Acta Psychiatr Scand 40:190–196, 1964.

19. Alfrey AC, Hegg A, Craswell P: Metabolism and toxicity of aluminum in renal failure. Am J Clin Nutr 33:1509–1516, 1980.

20. Arieff AI, Cooper JD, Armstrong D, Lazarowitz VC: Dementia, renal failure and brain aluminum. Ann Intern Med 90:741–747, 1979.

21. Kaehny WD, Hegg AP, Alfrey AC: Gastrointestinal absorption of aluminum from aluminum-containing antacids. New Engl J Med 296:1289–1390, 1977.

22. Benn A, Swan CJH, Cooke WT, et al.: Effect on intraluminal pH on the absorption of pteroylmonoglutamic acid. Br Med J 16:148–150, 1971.

23. Perry J, Chanarin I: Observations on folate absorption with particular reference to folate polyglutamate and possible inhibitors to its absorption. Gut 13:544–550, 1972.

24. MacKenzie JF, Russell RJ: The effect of pH on folic acid absorption. Clin Sci Molec Med 51:363–368, 1976.

25. Halsted CH: Intestinal absorption and malabsorption of folates. Ann Rev Med 31: 79–87, 1980.

26. Blair JA, Lucas ML, Swanston-Flatt SK: Intestinal folic acid absorption and the acid microclimate: The effects of compounds relevant to folate malabsorption. Phlugors Arch 392:20–33, 1981.

27. Fingl E, Freston JW: Antidiarrheal agents and laxatives: Changing concepts. Clin Gastroenterol 8:161–185, 1979.

28. Ganginella TS, Phillips SF: Ricinoleic acid: Current view of an ancient oil. Am J Dig Dis 20:1171–1177, 1975.

29. Donowitz M, Binder HJ: Effect of dioctyl sulfosuccinate on colonic fluid and electrolyte movement. Gastroenterology 69:941–950, 1975.

30. Hardcastle JD, Wilkins JL: The action of sennosides and related compounds on human colon and rectum. Gut 11:1038–1042, 1970.

31. Harvey RF, Read AE: Effects of oral magnesium sulfate on colonic motility in patients with the irritable bowel syndrome. Gut 14:983–987, 1973.

32. Harvey RF, Read AE: Mode of action of the saline purgatives. Am Heart J 89:810–812, 1975.

33. Fingl E: Laxatives and cathartics. In Goodman LS, Gilman A (eds): The Pharmacological Basis of Therapeutics, 5th ed. New York, Macmillan, 1975, p 978.

34. Brodribb AJM: Treatment of symptomatic diverticular disease with a high-fibre diet. Lancet 1:664–666, 1977.

35. Smith RG, Rowe MJ, Smith AN, et al.: A study of bulking agents in elderly patients. Age and Ageing 9:267–271, 1980.

36. Roe DA: Geriatric Nutrition. Englewood Cliffs, NJ, Prentice-Hall, 1983.

37. Fleming BJ, Genuth SM, Gould AB, Kaminokowski MD: Laxative-induced hypokalemia, sodium depletion and hyperreninemia: Effects of potassium and sodium replacement on the renin-angiotensin-aldosterone system. Ann Intern Med 83:60–62, 1975.

38. Levine D, Good EAW, Wingate DL: Purgative abuse associated with reversible cachexia, hypogammaglobulinemia, and finger clubbing. Lancet 1:919–920, 1981.

39. Frame B, Guiang HL, Frost HM, Reynolds WA: Osteomalacia induced by laxative (phenolphthalein) ingestion. Arch Intern Med 128:794–796, 1971.

40. Heizer WD, Warshaw AL, Waldmann TA, Laster L: Protein-losing gastroenteropathy and malabsorption associated with factitious diarrhea. Arch Intern Med 68:839–851, 1968.

41. Roe DA: Drug-Induced Nutritional Deficiencies. Westport, Conn, AVI Publishing, 1976, pp 130–132.

42. Burrows MT, Far WK: The action of mineral oil per os on the organism. Proc Soc Exp Biol Med 24:719–723, 1927.

43. Smith MC, Spector H: Calcium and phosphorus metabolism in rats and dogs as influenced by the ingestion of mineral oil. J Nutr 20:19–30, 1940.

44. Smith MC, Spector H: Some effects on animal nutrition of the ingestion of mineral oil. Univ Arizona Coll Agric Exp Sta Bull 84:373–395, 1940.

45. Javert CT, Marci C: Prothrombin concentration and mineral oil. J Obstet Gynecol 42:409–414, 1941.

46. Curtis AC, Ballmer RS: The prevention of carotene absorption by liquid petrolatum. JAMA 113:1795–1788, 1939.

47. Meulengracht E: Osteomalacia of the spinal column from deficient diet or from disease of the digestive tract. 3. Osteomalacia e abuse laxantium. Acta Med Scand 101:187–210, 1939.

48. Benson TA: Gastrointestinal reactions to drugs. Am J Dig Dis 16:357–362, 1971.

49. Dick WC, Buchanan WW: Advances in the treatment of rheumatic disorders. Practitioner 207:483–491, 1971.

50. Watson Buchanan W, Rooney PJ, Rennie AN: Aspirin and the salicylates. Clin Rheum Dis 5:499–537, 1979.
51. Hellon RF: Monamines, pyrogens and cations: Their actions on central control of body temperature. Pharmacol Rev 26:289–321, 1975.
52. Harrison MJG, Marshall J, Meadows JC, Russell RW: Effect of aspirin in amaurosis fugax. Lancet 2:743–744, 1981.
53. Jick H, Miettinen OS: Regular aspirin use and myocardial infarction. Br Med J 1:1057, 1976.
54. Leonards JH, Levy G: Gastrointestinal blood loss during prolonged aspirin administration. New Engl J Med 289:1020, 1973.
55. Quick AJ: Salicylates and bleeding: The aspirin tolerance test. Am J Med Sci 252:265–269, 1966.
56. Gouf KR, McCarthy C, Read AE, et al.: Folic acid deficiency in rheumatoid arthritis. Br. Med J 1:212–216, 1964.
57. Alter HJ, Zvaifler NJ, Rath CE: Interrelationship of rheumatoid arthritis, folic acid and aspirin. Blood 38:405–416, 1971.
58. Knapp, M: Analgesic nephropathy. Ann Intern Med 142:1197–1198, 1982.
59. Roe DA: Alcohol and the Diet. Westport, Conn, AVI Publishing, 1979.
60. Martin DC, Mead K: Reducing medication errors in a geriatric population. J Am Geriat Soc 30:258–260, 1981.

8 | Vitamin Use and Abuse Among The Elderly

Daphne A. Roe

Surveys of drug use among the elderly have shown that vitamin supplements figure among the most common "drugs" taken. In such surveys, vitamin preparations are not only among the principal drug groups prescribed, but also figure prominently among types of self-medication.[1]

Our goal is to explore indications for prescription of supplementary vitamins for elderly patients and the justifications that elderly people choose to explain their self-prescribed intake of such nutrient supplements. A further objective is to examine the efficacy and safety of these products.

EFFECT OF AGE AND RELATED HEALTH PROBLEMS ON VITAMIN REQUIREMENTS

It has been demonstrated that food energy requirements decline with age due to changes in metabolic rate and also to diminished physical activity.[2] At the same time, available data indicate that vitamin requirements do not change substantially as people get older.[3] It is for these reasons that a diet of high nutrient density is recommended for men and women of 65 years and older.[4] Among healthy elderly not showing clinical or biochemical evidence of vitamin deficiencies, it is generally assumed that they have successfully adjusted their vitamin intakes to meet their needs. However, in special groups of elderly, low intakes of dietary vitamins have been reported. Particularly low intakes of fat-soluble and water-soluble vitamins have been reported in institutionalized patients and in independently living elderly in the five years prior to death.[4-6]

Disabled elderly living outside institutions may find it easier to subsist on cookies and other foods of low vitamin content because these foods require neither preparation nor chewing. Studies by Carl[7] of the food purchases of homebound elderly show an association between the number of foods purchased and the vitamin content available from food. These studies suggest that elderly subsisting on a monotonous diet consisting of few foods are more at risk for the development of vitamin deficiencies.

Studies of vitamin absorption by older persons do not suggest an age-related decrement in absorptive capacity. When vitamin malabsorption is found in the elderly, it is related either to the presence of gastrointestinal disease, alcohol abuse, or intake of drugs that interfere with the absorption of these nutrients.[8-10]

Whereas we acknowledge that there are several risk factors for the development of avitaminoses among the elderly, surveys of independently living elderly do not demonstrate a high prevalence of vitamin deficiencies. Avitaminoses are also uncommon in hospitalized patients except in those who have diseases that severely limit nutrient intake, cause malabsorption, or impair vitamin utilization. On the basis of these findings, it is fair to assume that most elderly meet their vitamin needs either by consuming foods of adequate vitamin content and availability or by taking vitamin supplements.

RATIONAL PRESCRIPTION OF VITAMIN SUPPLEMENTS

Justifiable reasons for vitamin administration in the elderly include the treatment of avitaminoses or the prevention of avitaminoses in patients who are vitamin depleted due to diet, disease, or drug therapies. Vitamins may be appropriately

Table 8-1. Indications for Vitamin Administration in the Elderly

1. Risk factor(s) for vitamin depletion/deficiency present:
   a. Diet low in one or more vitamins
   b. Laboratory evidence of hypovitaminosis
   c. Malabsorption syndrome
   d. Alcohol abuse
   e. Intake of prescription or OTC drug known to impair vitamin status
2. Avitaminosis has been confirmed:
   a. Clinical diagnosis
   b. Biochemical tests for vitamin status in deficiency range
   c. Positive ancillary hematological or radiological tests
3. Vitamin dependency state is present, justifying need for pharmacological dose(s) of single vitamin:
   a. Wernicke's encephalophathy
   b. Intake of vitamin antagonist drug(s)*

* Justification of high-dose vitamin therapy depends on knowledge that the vitamin does not reduce drug efficacy.

used in the treatment of specific conditions that respond to single vitamins used as therapeutic agents (Table 8-1). When pharmacological doses of vitamins are used in the treatment of disease, this therapeutic approach can only be justified when efficacy has been proven by controlled clinical trials and follow-up studies upholding the original observations.

VITAMIN PRESCRIPTION WITHOUT PROOF OF EFFICACY

There are certain organic brain syndromes in the elderly that are appropriately treated by administration of specific vitamins. The most important of these is Wernicke's encephalopathy, which is a thiamin-dependent syndrome occurring mainly in alcoholics during drinking sprees. Wallace et al.[11] noted in a group of patients with Wernicke's syndrome who were in coma that all shared a history of alcoholism, previous alcoholic neurological disease, and poor nutrition. Intravenous or nasogastric tube feeding without vitamin supplements precipitated coma in three out of four of these patients. Three out of four of these patients died, perhaps in part because the cause of coma was not discovered early enough for appropriate high-dosage thiamin therapy.

Frequently, claims for the efficacy of specific vitamins in the control of chronic diseases of the elderly have not been substantiated by controlled studies. For example, when methenamine salts were first recommended for the prophylaxis of urinary tract infections in institutionalized elderly patients or in those with indwelling Foley catheters, it was recommended that ascorbic acid should be given concurrently to acidify the urine.[12-14] The efficacy of ascorbic acid for acidifying the urine has since been placed in doubt. Whereas McDonald and Murphy[15] found that 2.5 g daily of ascorbic acid given orally in fractional doses every four hours was adequate to obtain a urinary pH equal to or less than 5.5, Travis et al.[16] reported a variable effect on reduction of urinary pH with dosages of ascorbic acid of 2–4 g/day. These latter authors found that reduction in urinary pH was more consistent when ascorbic acid was given at dosages of 6–8 g/day.

A study was made by Nakarto et al.[17] of 73 elderly patients receiving methenamine and ascorbic acid concurrently. Urinary pH was assessed in relation to the dosage of ascorbic acid, duration of therapy, formulation, and dosing intervals for ascorbic acid and methenamine. Statistical analysis revealed a significant increase in urinary pH when the dose of ascorbic acid was increased. No significant relationship was found between urinary pH and the dosage forms of ascorbic acid, the salt of methenamine, or the duration of methenamine therapy. Changes in urinary pH at different dosing intervals of ascorbic acid were found only to be significant at the 10% level for the three-times-a-day daily dosage schedule. It therefore seems questionable whether ascorbic acid should appropriately be used to acidify the urine of catheterized patients receiving methenamine treatment.

Many elderly are given injections or oral doses of vitamin B_{12} by their physicians for appetite promotion. However, Herbert[18] has commented that every objective study demonstrates that vitamin B_{12} has no appetite-stimulant effect and has no effect on neurological disorders other than those due to vitamin B_{12} deficiency. There is one possible exception, that of tobacco amblyopia.

The administration of pharmacological doses of vitamins has been advocated by certain nutritionists who justify this practice on the basis of "latent vitamin deficits." Baker et al.[19] believe that elderly people often have vitamin deficiencies due to malabsorption. In a study of elderly persons living in a geriatric center, they found that 39% showed abnormal biochemical tests of nutritional status, which they believed indicated vitamin deficits. These "deficits" were present despite the fact that these patients were taking oral multivitamin supplements. When single intramuscular injections of multivitamins were given, these "deficits" were no longer detectable.

Since the biochemical parameters used to assess vitamin status of the elderly persons included in this study were not functional tests, it is somewhat difficult to assess or interpret the changes brought about by injection of the vitamins.

Advocates of vitamin therapy for the elderly may base their practices on findings of an association between subclinical vitamin deficiency and the presence of specific chronic disease in geriatric patients. For example, it has been shown in several studies that among elderly in geriatric care facilities, those with dementias are more likely to have low-folate status than those without such organic brain syndromes.[20-22] Sneath et al.,[23] who were among those who made the observation of impaired folate status being more common in elderly with dementias, believed that the most likely explanation for this finding is that dementia leads to poor dietary intake of folate and, hence, a folate deficiency. However, they considered the possibility that folate deficiency was associated with the decline in mental function and could not be excluded on the basis of then-current knowledge. There is, however, no well-controlled study indicating that administration of folic acid to elderly patients with dementia leads to an improvement in mental status. Vitamins are sometimes inappropriately prescribed because of one or more false concepts by physicians about indications for vitamin usage, as shown in Table 8-2.

EXTERNAL FACTORS INFLUENCING VITAMIN SELF-MEDICATION

It is rather generally held that elderly people are prone to take vitamins because they are susceptible to media claims. Although this may sometimes be the case, in the 1969 study of U.S. health practices and opinions carried out by the National Technical Information Service for the Food and Drug Administration,[24] it was found that vitamin users among the elderly as well as those in younger age groups cited physicians and pharmacists as their main source of influence for usage of these nutrient supplements.

However, in this same report, there is indication from responses to the questionnaire that vitamin users tend to believe that intake of these nutrient supplements can ameliorate symptoms that may accompany diseases common among the

Table 8-2. Determinants of Inappropriate Vitamin Prescription by Physicians

 1. General lack of nutrition knowledge
 2. False belief that vitamin requirements are increased by aging
 3. Conviction that aging or disease of the elderly is prevented by vitamins
 4. Lack of specific therapy for disease(s) present
 5. Erroneous belief that previous cures or palliation was due to vitamin therapy
 6. Request for vitamins by patient or family member
 7. Vitamin use is routine practice at the geriatric facility
 8. Incorrect belief that vitamins can increase patient's sense of well-being
 9. False conviction that patient's vitamin intake is low
10. Placebo effect

elderly. They may also believe that vitamins can prevent, or be used to treat, arthritis and cancer. In certain studies, it has been shown that vitamin preparations are among the most common over-the-counter drugs purchased. Chaiton et al.,[25] who obtained this finding, also observed that vitamin usage was reported to be the result of a physician's recommendation. It would be interesting to know whether the cited physician's recommendation for older patients to take vitamins is often real or more often imagined, or an exaggeration of the physician's assent to the patient's statement of need.

No consistent relationship between vitamin usage and age was found either in the FDA survey, the Chaiton investigation, or in an unpublished study conducted by the author of the demographic characteristics of persons who are users of over-the-counter drugs. Self-medication with vitamins in the elderly is attributable to factors indicated in Table 8-3.

NUTRIENT TOXICITY WITH EXCESSIVE INTAKE OF VITAMINS

Vitamin A

High-dosage vitamin A intake may be prescribed for the treatment of chronic dermatoses occurring among the elderly even though skin signs of vitamin A deficiency are very rare.[26] However, much more commonly, vitamin A is ingested to excess as self-medication. Symptoms of hypervitaminosis A are often misdiagnosed, particularly among the elderly, although the clinical features of this syn-

Table 8-3. Determinants of Over-the-Counter Vitamin Use by the Elderly

1. Belief in prevention of aging and age-related disease by vitamin
2. Media or company claims for reversal of memory loss by vitamin
3. M.D. has failed to alleviate health problems present by drugs
4. Advice by pharmacist
5. Advice of friends or family
6. Advice by M.D.
7. Concern that diet is vitamin deficient
8. Conversion to health foods and natural vitamin usage

drome have been clearly described in older persons. Hypervitaminosis A in adults is manifested by xeroderma, partial alopecia with loss of the hair of the eyebrows, anorexia, and headaches.[27] Bone pains, visual disturbances, and a hemorrhagic diathesis with epistaxis and bleeding gums may also be encountered.[28]

Total doses of vitamin A that have caused signs of intoxication are in the order of 150,000 to 200,000 international units (IU). It has been noted, however, that vitamin A intoxication tends to occur with continued high-dosage vitamin A therapy over a period of several months up to several years.[29] More rarely, chronic hypervitaminosis A can result in hepatic damage with portal hypertension and ascites. Clinically, this syndrome closely resembles alcoholic cirrhosis. Skin changes are those of vitamin A intoxication.[30]

Liver damage associated with vitamin A intoxication in older people may not be reversible by withdrawal of the vitamin. Garry[31] has indicated that suspicion of vitamin A intoxication is a clear justification for biochemical assessment of vitamin A status. The best method for biochemical assessment of vitamin A status in these persons is by high-performance liquid chromatography separation of retinol and retinyl esters in the plasma. It is only with vitamin A intoxication that significant amounts of retinyl esters appear in the plasma.

Vitamin D

Vitamin D intoxication is no longer common among the elderly because of restricted over-the-counter sales. However, it is still possible for the public to purchase bottles of vitamin D (400 IU) tablets, and if large numbers of these are consumed, vitamin D toxicity will result. The signs of vitamin D overdosage include anorexia, nausea, vomiting, thirst, constipation, sometimes fever, abdominal pain, pallor, fatigue, and diarrhea, as well as signs of renal damage and radiological evidence of metastatic calcification.

In the elderly, signs of vitamin D intoxication may cause an organic brain syndrome. Two cases of vitamin D intoxication occurring in elderly people were reported by Verner et al.[32] In both cases, vitamin D had been sold to patients without prescription, and by the time they were admitted to a hospital, they were mentally disoriented and could not remember taking the vitamins. In the first case, a 71-year-old man was found to have taken 200,000 IU of vitamin D per day for a month. In the second case, a 69-year-old woman was discovered to have taken 300,000 IU of vitamin D a day intermittently for a period of three years. The diagnosis was made on the basis of clinical signs and laboratory findings and only later corroborated by the pharmacist's report. Neither case was fatal, although the woman showed some evidence of renal damage after a two-year follow-up period.

Evidence has been obtained that in vitamin D intoxication the metabolite responsible is 25-hydroxycholecalciferol. This hypothesis is supported by the demonstration that patients who are anephric and therefore incapable of synthesizing 1,25-dihydroxycholecalciferol can become vitamin D intoxicated.[33,34]

On the other hand, in a study by Lund et al.[35] of the effects of treatment of osteoporosis among the elderly with alpha-hydroxycholecalciferol for three to four months, it was shown that hypercalcemia can result, indicating routine treatment of osteoporosis in the elderly by this vitamin D metabolite could be dangerous.

Vitamin E

Megadoses of vitamin E have been claimed to cause coagulation defects in patients receiving coumarin antagonists. Suggestion has been made that the metabolites of alpha-tocopherol that occur in the body, such as alpha-tocopheryl quinone or hydroquinone, may act as antimetabolites to vitamin K.[36]

Niacin

The side effects induced by high-dosage niacin therapy include not only the well-known flush, but also impaired hepatic function and a number of dermatological side effects, including pruritus, desquamation, and acanthosis nigricans–like lesions.[37]

Niacin is included in tonics for the elderly for which a false claim is made of cerebral vasodilatation and improvement in memory.

Vitamin C

Elderly people who have cancer may take megadoses of vitamin C in the mistaken belief that this vitamin can promote cure.[38] Serious side effects are uncommon, but "gas pain" and diarrhea may occur, as well as burning on urination. Further, high vitamin C intake for prolonged periods can accelerate the formation of oxalate stones.

Symptoms and signs of hypervitaminoses are summarized in Table 8-4.

VITAMIN INTERFERENCE WITH DRUG EFFICACY

Pharmacological doses of vitamins can reduce the blood levels of certain drugs and reduce the desired therapeutic effect. High doses of folic acid or vitamin B_6 given to patients receiving phenytoin and/or phenobarbital for seizure disorders can reduce blood levels of these drugs and thereby reduce their therapeutic efficacy.[39-41]

Recently, cases of warfarin resistance have been reported due to intake of vitamin K in liquid nutrient supplements.[42] Lee et al.[43] reported on a 70-year-old woman who had had a pelvic exenteration for carcinoma of the proximal urethra. In the next three weeks, she received a crystalline amino acid solution without vitamin K supplementation and a 14-day course of chloramphenicol for treatment of a *Bacteroides fragilis* septicemia. During her convalescence, she developed a deep venous thrombosis that was managed with heparin. From day seven to day ten of the heparin treatment, warfarin therapy was initiated and continued at a dosage of 10 mg/day. Prothrombin time did not increase in response to warfarin administration, and it

Table 8-4. Clinical Features of Hypervitaminoses in the Elderly

Vitamin	Acute Effect of Pharmacological Dose	Signs and Symptoms of Chronic Vitamin Overload
Vitamin A	—	Dry skin, partial alopecia, loss of eyebrows, anorexia, headache, bone pain, jaundice, hepatomegaly, ascites
Vitamin D	Anorexia	Headache, confusion, polyuria, hypercalcemia, uremia
Vitamin E	—	Decreased prothrombin levels, purpura (in patients on coumarin anticoagulants)
Niacin	Flushing	Hepatic dysfunction, hyperglycemia, peptic ulcer, acanthosis nigricans
Vitamin C	Gas, diarrhea, burning on urination	Accelerated formation of renal calculi (oxalate)

was subsequently discovered that the patient had been receiving three cans of Ensure per day for seven days, which contributed 0.72 mg of vitamin to her vitamin K intake. When her nutrient supplement was changed to Meritene, which contains only trace amounts of vitamin K, her prothrombin time fell to reach the therapeutic range on daily doses of 5 mg/day of warfarin. The authors of this report have supplied a list of nutrient supplements with their vitamin K contents. A revised version of this list, which includes vitamin preparations, is shown in Table 8-5. It should be useful to physicians working with, or caring for, elderly patients who are on coumarin anticoagulants.

CHARACTERISTICS OF VITAMIN USERS AND NONUSERS

The vitamin usage rate among the elderly has been reported as being between 35% and 75% of respondents.[44-49] According to Read and Graney,[1] characteristics of nonusers are that they find they have no need to take vitamins, they don't believe in taking vitamins, they feel well, or the vitamins cost too much. These authors, in keeping with previous authors, report that vitamin users cite medical advice as a major reason for taking vitamins. Other reasons include a need for bone strength, for which it is believed that vitamins, as well as minerals, may be taken, and the prevention of colds, for which vitamins C and E are taken. Vitamin users are also more likely than nonusers to state that they feel themselves to be in poor health.

There are, however, several other major categories of elderly vitamin users. There are those who have a disease that does not respond to vitamin therapy. Included in this category are people previously discussed who have defined avitaminoses and those with vitamin dependency syndromes, such as the Wernicke-

Table 8-5. Vitamin K Content of Nutrition Products and Vitamin Mixtures Taken by Geriatric Patients

Product Name	Manufacturer	Vitamin K μg/1000 Cal
Nutri-1000 LF	Cutter	150
Vipep	Cutter	75
Compleat B (cans)	Doyle	25[a]
Meritene	Doyle	trace
Precision-HN	Doyle	33
Precision-Isotonic	Doyle	64
Precision-LR	Doyle	53
Vivonex	Eaton	22
Vivonex-HN	Eaton	22
Amin-Aid	McGaw	0
Hepatic-Aid	McGaw	0
Flexical	Mead Johnson	125
Isocal	Mead Johnson	125
Nutramigen	Mead Johnson	719
Portagen	Mead Johnson	737
Pregestimil	Mead Johnson	710
Prosobee	Mead Johnson	156
Sustacal	Mead Johnson	235
Magnacal	Organon	0[b]
Renu	Organon	0[b]
Vitaneed	Organon	0[b]
Ensure	Ross	943 (146)[c]
Ensure-Plus	Ross	1060 (208)[c]
Isomil	Ross	220 (150)[c]
Osmolite	Ross	943 (146)[c]
Vital	Ross	1330 (186)[c]
Neo Mull Soy	Syntex	78
Chlorophyll Complex (perles)	Standard Process	3.3 mg (6 perles)[d]
Total Formula	Vitaline Formulas	79 (1 tab)[d]
SynKayvite	Roche	5–10 mg (1–2 tabs)[d]

[a] Doyle planned to increase vitamin K content by January 1981.

[b] Organon planned to increase vitamin K content of formulation by January 1981.

[c] Current vitamin K_1 content/1000 Kcal in parentheses.

[d] Recommended daily dose

Adapted from Lee M, Schwartz RN, and Sharifi R: Warfarin resistance and vitamin K. Ann Intern Med 94:140–141, 1981.

Korsakoff syndrome. There are also those elderly men and women who have recently experienced vitamin depletion due to dietary restriction, vitamin-free IV therapy, and/or drug administration. A larger group consists of those persons who incorrectly believe in the efficacy of vitamins as palliative or curative agents for their presenting health problems. These include sufferers from severe arthritis and, less commonly, those with chronic cardiovascular disease or neurological disease. Finally, there are the patients of physicians who prescribe vitamins inappropriately for a variety of ailments, either knowing that the vitamins are placebos, or because of some mistaken idea about the physiological or pharmacological properties of these agents.

REFERENCES

1. Read MH, Graney AS: Food supplement usage by the elderly. J Am Diet Assoc 80:250–253, 1982.
2. Shock NW: Energy metabolism, caloric intake and physical activity in aging. In Carlson LA (ed): Nutrition in Old Age. Uppsala, Almqvist & Wiksell, 1972, p 12.
3. Munro HN: Introduction to minisymposium on nutrition and aging. In Harper AE, Davis GK (eds): Nutrition in Health and Disease and International Development. International Congress on Nutrition. New York, Alan R Liss, 1981, pp 677–685.
4. Schlenker ED, Feurig JS, Stone JH, et al.: Nutrition and health in older people. Am J Clin Nutr 26:1111–1119, 1973.
5. Kelley L, Ohlson MA, Harper LJ: Food selection and well-being of aging women. J Am Diet Assoc 33:466–467, 1957.
6. Chope HD: Relation of nutrition to health in aging persons: A four-year follow-up of a study in San Mateo County. Calif Med 81:335–338, 1954.
7. Carl JW: Food purchases of housebound elderly. M.N.S. thesis. Ithaca, Cornell University, 1980.
8. Isselbacher K: Malabsorption syndromes including disease of pancreatic and biliary origin. In Winick N (ed): Nutrition and Gastroenterology. New York, Wiley, 1980, pp 93–104.
9. Mezey E: Intestinal function in chronic alcoholism. Ann New York Acad Sci 252:215–227, 1975.
10. Roe DA: Drug-nutrient interrelationships. Pract Gastroenterol 6:32–38, 1982.
11. Wallace WE, Willoughby E, Baker P: Coma in the Wernicke-Korsakoff syndrome. Lancet 3:400–401, 1978.
12. Hamilton-Miller JMT, Brumfitt W: Methenamine and its salts as urinary tract antiseptics: Variables affecting the antibacterial activity of formaldehyde, mandelic acid and hippuric acid in vitro. Invest Urol 14:287–291, 1977.
13. Gandelman AL: Methenamine mandelate: Antimicrobial activity in urine and correlation with formaldehyde levels. J Urol 97:533–536, 1967.
14. Musher DM, Griffith DP: Generation of formaldehyde from methenamine: Effect of pH and concentration and antibacterial effect. Antimicrob Agents Chemother 6:708–711, 1974.
15. McDonald DF, Murphy GP: Bacteriostatic and acidifying effects of methenamine, hydrolized casein and ascorbic acid on the urine. New Eng J Med 261:803, 1959.
16. Travis LB, Dodge WF, Mintz AA, Assemi M: Urinary acidification with ascorbic acid. J Pediat 67:1176–1178, 1965.
17. Nakarto DV, Bell CJ, Lamy PP: Appraisal of ascorbic acid for acidifying the urine of methenamine-treated geriatric patients. J Am Geriat Soc 27:34–37, 1979.
18. Herbert V: Megavitamin therapy. In Contemporary Nutrition II. 1, 2, 1977. Reprinted in LaBuza TP, Sloan AE (eds): Contemporary Nutrition Controversies, St. Paul and New York, West Publishing, 1979, pp 223–227.
19. Baker H, Frank O, Jaslow SP: Oral versus intramuscular vitamin supplementation for hypovitaminoses in the elderly. J Am Geriat Soc 28:42–46, 1980.
20. Jensen ON, Olesen OV: Folic acid concentrations in psychiatric patients. Acta Psychol Scand 45:289–294, 1969.
21. Kariks J, Perry SW: Folic acid deficiency in psychiatric patients. Med J Aust 1A:1192, 1195, 1970.
22. Hunter R, Jones M, Jones TG, Matthews DM: Serum B_{12} and folate concentrations in mental patients. Br J Psychiat 113:1291–1295, 1967.
23. Sneath P, Chanarin I, Hodkinson HM, et al.: Folate status in a geriatric population and

its relation to dementia. Age and Ageing 2:177–181, 1973.

24. National Technical Information Service. A study of health practices and opinions: Final report. FDA/DHEW Contract FDA 66–193, June 1972.

25. Chaiton A, Spitzer WO, Roberts RS, Delmore T: Patterns of medical drug use: A community focus. Can Med Assoc J 114:33–37, 1976.

26. Verbov J: Skin Diseases in the Elderly. London: Heinemann Medical Books, Ltd, 1974, p 172.

27. Bergen SS Jr, Roels OA: Hypervitaminosis A: Report of a case. Am J Clin Nutr 16:265–269, 1965.

28. Creek DW, McNiece KJ, Nelson LM: Hypervitaminosis A: Toxic reaction. Am J Gastroenterol 29:169–172, 1958.

29. Roe DA: Nutrient toxicity with excessive intake. 1. Vitamins. NY State J Med 66:869–873, 1966.

30. Russell RM, Boyer JL, Bagheri SA, Hruban Z: Hepatic injury from chronic hypervitaminosis A resulting in portal hypertension and ascites. New Eng J Med 291:435–440, 1974.

31. Garry PJ: Vitamin A. Clinics in Lab Med 1:699–711, 1981.

32. Verner JV Jr, Engel FL, McPherson HT: Vitamin D intoxication: Report of 2 cases treated with cortisone. Ann Intern Med 48:765–773, 1958.

33. Haussler MR, McCain TA: Basic and clinical concepts related to vitamin D metabolism in action. New Eng J Med 297:1041–1050, 1977.

34. Counts SJ, Baylink DJ, Shen FH, et al.: Vitamin D intoxication in an anephric child. Ann Intern Med 82:196–200, 1975.

35. Lund B, Hjorth L, Kjaer I, et al.: Treatment of osteoporosis of aging with 1-alpha-hydroxy-cholecalciferol. Lancet 2:1168–1171, 1975.

36. Arnrich L: Toxic effects of megadoses of fat-soluble vitamins. In Hathcock JN, Coon J (eds) Nutrition and Drug Interrelations. New York, Academic Press, 1978, pp 751–771.

37. Roe DA: Cutaneous effects of hypocholesterolemic agents. NY State J Med 64:2559–2563, 1964.

38. DiPalma JR, McMichael R: Assessing the value of meganutrients in disease. Bull NY Acad Med 58:254–262, 1982.

39. Baylis EM, Crowley JM, Preece JM, et al.: Influence of folic acid on blood phenytoin levels. Lancet 1:62–64, 1971.

40. Mattson RA, Gallagher BB, Reynolds GH, Glass D: Folate therapy in epilepsy: A controlled study. Arch Neurol 29:78–81, 1971.

41. Roe DA: Drug-nutrient interactions. Med Clin N Am 63:985–1007, 1979.

42. Riley R, Rytand D: Resistance to warfarin due to unrecognized vitamin K supplementation. New Eng J Med 303:160–161, 1980.

43. Lee M, Schwartz RN, Sharifi R: Warfarin resistance and vitamin K. Ann Intern Med 94:140–141, 1981.

44. Harrill I, Cervone N: Vitamin status of older women. Am J Clin Nutr 30:431–440, 1977.

45. Dibble MV, Brin M, Thiele VF, et al.: Evaluation of nutritional status of elderly subjects with a comparison between fall and spring. J Am Geriat Soc 15:1031–1061, 1967.

46. Le Bovit C: The food of older persons living at home. J Am Diet Assoc 46:285–289, 1965.

47. Steinkamp RC, Cohen NL, Walsh HE: Resurvey of an aging population: 14 years follow-up. The San Mateo Nutrition Study. J Am Diet Assoc 46:103–110, 1965.

48. Davidson CS, Livermore J, Anderson R, Kaufman S: The nutrition of a group of apparently healthy ageing persons. Am J Clin Nutr 10:181–199, 1962.

49. McGandy RB, Barrows Ch Jr, Spanias A, et al.: Nutrient intakes and energy expenditure in men of different ages. J Gerontol 21:581–587, 1966.

Index